MRCP PART 2

A Revision for the
New Format of the Written Section

MRCP PART 2
A Revision for the New Format of the Written Section

Farhad U Huwez
MB ChB, PhD (Glasgow), MRCPI, FRCP
(Glasgow and London)
Consultant Physician
Basildon University Hospital
Nethermayne, Basildon
Essex, UK

Udayaraj Umasankar
MB BS, DTRD, MRCP (UK)
Specialist Medical Registrar
University Hospital Lewisham
Lewisham, London,
UK

Christopher Ah Wah Chan
MB BCh, MD (Wales), FRCP (Glasgow and London)
Consultant Physician
Clacton and District Hospital and
Colchester General Hospital
Essex, UK

JAYPEE

JAYPEE BROTHERS MEDICAL PUBLISHERS
The Health Sciences Publisher
New Delhi | London

Jaypee Brothers Medical Publishers (P) Ltd

Headquarters
EMCA House, 23/23-B Ansari Road,
Daryaganj New Delhi 110 002, India
Landline: +91-11-23272143,
+91-11-23272703
+91-11-23282021, +91-11-23245672
e-mail: jaypee@jaypeebrothers.com

Corporate Office
4838/24, Ansari Road,
Daryaganj New Delhi 110 002, India
Phone: +91-11-43574357
Fax: +91-11-43574314
e-mail: jaypee@jaypeebrothers.com

Overseas Office
JP Medical Ltd.
83, Victoria Street, London
SW1H 0HW (UK)
Phone: +44-20 3170 8910
e-mail: info@jpmedpub.com

EU GPSR Authorised Representative
Logos Europe, 9 rue Nicolas Poussin
17000, La Rochelle, France
Phone: +33 (0) 6 67 93 73 78
e-mail: contact@logoseurope.eu

Website: www.jaypeebrothers.com
Website: www.jaypeedigital.com

MRCP PART 2
First Edition: 2007
Reprint: 2026
ISBN: 978-81-8061-910-6
Printed at: Samrat Offset Pvt. Ltd.

Dr Huwez Family (My Wife Abeer, My Children Tara and Mustafa and Memories of My Mother and Behistun)

Dr Umasankar Family (My Parents Mrs and Dr Udayaraj, My Wife Lakshmi and My Daughters Deekshitha and Deepti)

Dr Chan Family (My Parents, My Brother David and My Sisters Suzanne, Sally and Michelle)

'Real knowledge is to know the extent of one's ignorance.'

Confucius 551 - 479 BC

This is our second publication in a series of books designed to help postgraduate doctors who are taking the MRCP (UK) and other postgraduate diplomas in General (Internal) Medicine. In July 2002 a new type of written examination for the part 2 of the MRCP (UK) diploma was introduced and consisted of two papers, each of two and a half hours' duration, in which candidates have to select the most appropriate answer from 5 given possibilities ("best of five") or choose 2 or more from a longer list ("n from many"). In July 2004, this new format is extended so that each of the two written papers is three hours long and contain up to 90 questions (see www.mrcpuk.org for details).

The questions in this book are based on real cases and include common medical problems and emergencies, interesting rarities, and "topical" diseases taken from a large number of medical specialities. In our answers, we have summarised essential factual information and provided practical tips for future reference. Links to our previous book* have also been given. Many sections are reviewed by many of our colleagues and we are very grateful to them for their advice. Among those who helped specifically within their specialities include Dr Nagui Gendi, Consultant Rheumatologist at Basildon Hospital, Dr Dipak Mukherjee, Consultant in Respiratory Medicine at Basildon Hospital, and Dr. B. Vijayan, Specialist Registrar in Gastroenterology at Aberdeen Royal Infirmary in Scotland, and Dr U. P. Udayaraj, Specialist Registrar in Renal Medicine at Oxford, England. We are also especially grateful to Dr Richard Shen (Consultant physician in Genitourinary and HIV Medicine at Thurrock Primary Care NHS Trust) for his critical review of the cases on infectious diseases.

The discussions are also useful for the presentations in the clinical part of the MRCP (UK) PACES. We hope junior hospital doctors will enjoy using this book in their revision for the part 2 MRCP (UK) examination. We also hope this book and others in the series will help trainees acquire a good working knowledge of General (Internal) Medicine, which is an essential requirement before enrolment into higher specialist medical training. Clinical medicine is constantly evolving and changing and, therefore, for any future edition we would warmly welcome constructive comments on any of our clinical cases.

Farhad Huwez
Udayaraj Umasankar
Christopher Chan

*Book One: C. Chan, U. Umasankar and F. Huwez. Case Histories and Data Interpretation for MRCP Examinations. Jaypee Brothers Medical Publishers (P) Ltd, New Delhi, India. 2003. ISBN 81-8061-158-2.

'Unlike traditional questions in MRCP examination books, the "titles" of the cases give away the diagnosis or clues to the diagnosis. The format of MRCP examination question is maintained at the same time and the discussions have been made extensive so as to enable the reader to apply clinical knowledge on other questions related to the same topic. This is intended to keep the reader at ease with the book.'

Acknowledgements

The authors are extremely grateful to colleagues in the Medical Photography Department at Basildon University Hospital for their help in producing the illustrations.

List of Abbreviations

A and E	Accident and Emergency
ACE-I	Angiotensin Converting Enzyme Inhibitor
ACTH	Adrenocorticotrophic Hormone
ADH	Antidiuretic Hormone
AF	Atrial Fibrillation
ALP	Alkaline Phosphatase
ALT	Alanine Aminotransferase
ANA	Antinuclear Antibody
ANCA	Antineutrophilic Cytoplasmic Antibody
APTT	Activated Partial Thromboplastin Time
ARB	Angiotensin II Receptor Blocker
ARDS	Adult Respiratory Distress Syndrome
AST	Aspartate Aminotransferase
bd	*bis die* (twice daily)
BMI	Body Mass Index
BP	Blood Pressure
bpm	beats per minute
CCU	Coronary Care Unit
CK	Creatine Kinase
COPD	Chronic Obstructive Pulmonary Disease
CRP	C-Reactive Protein
CSF	Cerebrospinal Fluid
CT	Computed Tomography
CXR	Chest X-ray
DHAS	Dehydroepiandrosterone Sulphate
DLCO	Diffusion Capacity of Lung for Carbon Monoxide
DVT	Deep Venous Thrombosis
ECG	Electrocardiogram
ECHO	Echocardiogram
EEG	Electroencephalogram
e.g.	*exempli gratia* (for example)
ENT	Ear, Nose & Throat Department
EPO	Erythropoietin
ESR	Erythrocyte Sedimentation Rate
FEV1	Forced Expiratory Volume in one second

FEV%	Forced Expiratory Volume as per cent of Vital Capacity
FSH	Follicle Stimulating Hormone
FBC	Full Blood Count
FVC	Forced Vital Capacity
g-GT	Gamma-Glutamyl Transpeptidase
GH	Growth Hormone
GHRH	Growth Hormone Releasing Hormone
GTN	Glyceryl Trinitrate
Hb	Haemoglobin
HbA1c	Glycated haemoglobin
HCO3	Bicarbonate
HDL	High Density Lipoprotein
HDU	High Dependency Unit
IgG	Immunoglobulin G
IGF	Insulin Like Growth Factor
IgM	Immunoglobulin M
INR	International Normalised Ratio
ITU	Intensive Therapy Unit
IV	Intravenous
IVC	Inferior Vena Cava
KCO	Diffusion Constant (DLCO/VA)
KHz	Kilohertz
LFT	Liver Function Tests
LH	Luteinising Hormone
LVF	Left ventricular Failure
LVH	Left Ventricular Hypertrophy
mg	milligrams
mcg	micrograms
MCH	Mean Corpuscular Haemoglobin
MCHC	Mean Corpuscular Haemoglobin Concentration
MCV	Mean Corpuscular Volume
MI	Myocardial infarction
mmHg	millimetre of mercury
MRA	Magnetic Resonance Angiography
MRI	Magnetic Resonance Imaging
MSU	Mid Stream Urine
N.B.	*nota bene* (note well, or take notice)
NSAID	Non-steroidal Anti-inflammatory Drug
od	*omni die* (daily)

PaCO2	Partial pressure of carbon dioxide in arterial blood
PaO2	Partial pressure of oxygen in arterial blood
PCR	Polymerase Chain Reaction
PEFR	Peak Expiratory Flow Rate
PO4	Serum Phosphate
po	*per os* (by mouth)
PSA	Prostate Specific Antigen
PT	Prothrombin time
PTH	Parathyroid Hormone
qds	*quarter die sumendus* (four times daily)
RBBB	Right Bundle Branch Block
ref	Reference value (s)
RV	Residual Lung Volume
SIADH	Syndrome of Inappropriate ADH secretion
s/c	Subcutaneous
SaO2	Oxygen Saturation
SLE	Systemic Lupus Erythematosus
SSRI	Selective Serotonin Re-uptake Inhibitor
SVC	Static Vital Capacity
TB	Tuberculosis
TBG	Thyroid Binding Globulin
tds	*ter die sumendus* (three times daily)
TED	Thromboembolic Disease
TRH	Thyrotropin Releasing Hormone
TSH	Thyroid Stimulating Hormone
TLC	Total Lung Capacity
tPA	Tissue Plasminogen Activator
UFC	Urinary Free Cortisol
U and E	Urea and Electrolytes
VA	Alveolar Volume
VTE	Veno-thromboembolism
WBC	White Blood Cell count

Recommended International Non-Proprietary Name (rINN)

The European directive 92/27/EEC requires the use of Recommended International Non-proprietary Name (rINN) for medicinal substances. In most instances the British Approved Name (BAN) and the Recommended International Non-proprietary Name (rINN) differ slightly in spelling. A complete list of substances with proposed name changes is available from the British National Formulary website: *www.bnf.org.uk.* The following table gives the British Approved Name (BAN) and the Recommended International Non-proprietary Name (rINN) for some of the drugs quoted in this book. For the correct doses of all drugs and their approved name, please consult your local formulary.

BAN	*rINN*
adrenaline	epinephrine
amoxycillin	amoxicillin
amphetamine	amfetamine
bendrofluazide	bendroflumethiazide
busulphan	busulfan
cholestyramine	colestyramine
corticotrophin	corticotropin
cyclosporin	ciclosporin
dothiepin	dosulepin
frusemide	furosemide
hydroxyurea	hydroxycarbamide
noradrenaline	norepinephrine
oestradiol	estradiol
oxpentifylline	pentoxifylline
phenobarbitone	phenobarbital
thyroxine	levothyroxine
sulphasalazine	sulfasalazine

Internet Resources

The following websites provide an extensive catalogue of medical reviews. Basic information is provided by the online version of the Merck manual. In depth articles from Emedicine and Medscape are constantly updated. Bandolier provides succinct summaries of the latest evidence based medicine. Registered users of Medscape and Mdlinx receive regular emails that contain information on the latest articles selected from a wide range of medical journals. Registration is not always required and at present access to these sites is free of charge.

www.emedicine.com
www.medscape.com
www.postgradmed.com
www.mdlinx.com
www.merck.com/pubs/mmanual
www.jr2.ox.ac.uk/bandolier

The following websites provide up to date information on health care guidelines that are used in the UK:

www.nice.org.uk
www.bnf.org.uk
www.hyp.ac.uk/bhs/resources/guidelines.htm
www.dvla.gov.uk
www.rcplondon.ac.uk

General purpose search engine:
www.google.com

General medicine journal:
www.bmj.com

Handheld Computer Software Websites

The following websites provide free software for use in handheld computers, including medical calculators and patient tracking systems:

www.palmgear.com
www.memoware.com
www.handheldmed.com
http://5star.freeserve.com/PDA
www.handango.com

Each medical institution will have its own reference values. The following table is for guidance only

Normal Values in SI units

Aldosterone		100-800 pmol/l
Adrenocorticotrophic hormone	ACTH	10-80 ng/l
Alkaline phosphatase	ALP	35-130 U/l
Aminotransferase:	AST	10-40 U/l
(*or* transaminase)	ALT	5-40 U/l
Arterial blood gases (on air):	pH	7.35-7.45
	PaO_2	10-13 kPa
	$PaCO_2$	4.5-6.0 kPa
Bicarbonate	HCO_3	22-30 mmol/l
Bilirubin:	Total	3-17 μmol/l
	Conjugated	< 3.4 μmol/l
Calcitonin		< 11.5 ng/l
Calcium (corrected)	Ca	2.20-2.65 mmol/l
Chloride	Cl	95-105 μmol/l
Creatinine		60-120 μmol/l
Creatine kinase:	Men	30-220 U/l
	Women	20-170 U/l
Ferritin		20-300 μg/l
Folate:	Serum	5-40 nmol/l
	Red cell	770-1800 nmol/l
γ-glutamyl transpeptidase	γ-GT	7-32 U/l
Magnesium	Mg	0.7-1.1 mmol/l
Plasma osmolality		280-296 mosmol/kg
Phosphate	PO_4	0.8-1.4 mmol/l
Potassium	K	3.5-5.0 mmol/l
Prostate specific antigen	PSA	< 4 μg/l
Prolactin		< 600 mU/l
Protein:	Albumin	35-50 g/l
	Globulin	20-25 g/l

Parathyroid hormone	PTH	1.6-6.9 pmol/l
Renin		0.5-3.1 pmol/ml/hour
Sodium	Na	135-145 mmol/l
Thyroid peroxidase antibody	TPO	0-70 U/ml
Thyroglobulin		< 60 μg/l
Thyrotropin	TSH	0.4-5.0 mU/l
Total thyroxine	TT4	70-140 nmol/l
Free thyroxine	FT4	12.0-23.0 pmol/l
Total T3	TT3	1.2-3.0 nmol/l
Free T3	FT3	4.0-7.8 pmol/l
Urea		2.5-6.7 mmol/l
Total cholesterol		3.5-6.5 mmol/l (ideal < 5.0 mmol/l)
LDL cholesterol		1.5-4.4 mmol/l (ideal < 3.0 mmol/l)
HDL cholesterol:	Men	0.9-1.7 mmol/l (ideal > 1.0 mmol/l)
	Women	1.0-2.2 mmol/l (ideal > 1.0 mmol/l)
Triglycerides:	Men	0.7-2.2 mmol/l (ideal < 1.7 mmol/l)
	Women	0.6-1.7 mmol/l (ideal < 1.7 mmol/l)
Haemoglobin:	Men	14.0-17.7 g/dl
	Women	12.2-15.2 g/dl
WBC		4.0-10.0 × 10^9/l
Platelets		150-400 × 10^9/l
MCH		27-33 pg
MCHC		32-35 g/dl
MCV		80-96 fl
ESR		< 20 mm/h
Prothrombin time		10.7-13 seconds
Activated Partial Thromboplastin Time		25-33 seconds
Fibrin Degradation Products		< 5 μg/ml
D-dimers		< 0.5 μg/ml
Vitamin B_{12}		130-660 pmol/l
25(OH) vitamin D_3		20-110 nmol/l

Urinary calcium	2.5-7.5 mmol/day
Urinary free cortisol	50-180 nmol/day
Urinary 5HIAA	< 50 µmol/day
Urinary free epinephrine	20-110 nmol/day
Urinary norepinephrine	100-560 nmol/day

Numerical Abbreviations

Abbreviation	*Symbol*	*Value*		*Example*	
deci	d	10^{-1}	1/10	dl	decilitre
centi	c	10^{-2}	1/100	cm	centimetre
milli	m	10^{-3}	1/1,000	mmol	millimole
micro	ì	10^{-6}	1/1,000,000	ìmol	micromole
nano	n	10^{-9}	1/1,000,000,000	nmol	nanomole
pico	p	10^{-12}	1/1,000,000,000,000	pmol	picomole
femto	f	10^{-15}	1/1,000,000,000,000,000	fl	femtolitre

List of Cases

Case 1

Hypopituitarism

A 60-year-old woman was found unconscious at home. She had pituitary surgery and radiotherapy 3 years earlier for acromegaly. The neighbours noticed she was irritable in the last three days. She smoked heavily. No drug history was available on admission. She looked pale, the extremities were cold and the rectal temperature was 36° Celsius. Her blood pressure was 96/56 mm Hg. Biochemical screen showed:

Na	112 mmol/l
K	5.7 mmol/l
Urea	2.0 mmol/l
Glucose	2.0 mmol/l

What is the most likely underlying pathology?

A. Primary hypothyroidism
B. Primary hypoadrenalism
C. Hypopituitarism
D. Syndrome of inappropriate ADH secretion
E. Dilutional hyponatraemia

Answer (C)

DISCUSSION

Hypopituitarism

In the context of previous pituitary surgery and radiotherapy, the most likely diagnosis is hypopituitarism with ACTH deficiency (secondary adrenal failure) and TSH deficiency (secondary hypothyroidism). Radiation damage to the hypothalamus causes the gradual onset of anterior pituitary hormone deficiency. Generally, growth hormone deficiency is the first to appear, being followed by failure of gonadotrophin, ACTH and then TSH, but posterior pituitary hormone production is only rarely affected.

In this patient hypothyroidism impairs the ability to excrete a water load. Hyponatraemia, hyperkalaemia and hypoglycaemia indicate adrenal failure secondary to pituitary ACTH deficiency. The initial therapeutic measures are intravenous hydrocortisone, normal saline and glucose. Levothyroxine is given after adequate corticosteroid treatment. Corticosteroid and levothyroxine replacement therapy will have to be life long. The patient will need to carry a steroid card and instructed to increase the dose of corticosteroid to cover any acute severe illness, trauma or surgery.

Causes of hypopituitarism

- Pituitary adenomas
- Primary tumours in the near vicinity of the pituitary: craniopharyngioma and meningioma.
- Pituitary metastases: secondary spread from breast and lung malignancy accounts for two-thirds of all pituitary metastases. Less common are pituitary metastases from cancer of the prostate, colon, and kidney.
- Pituitary haemorrhage and infarction (pituitary apoplexy), e.g. postpartum as in Sheehan's syndrome. This presents with headache, vomiting, meningeal irritation, cranial nerve palsy and visual loss.
- Infiltration and granulomas: sarcoidosis, haemochromatosis, histiocytosis, Wegener's granulomatosis and lymphocytic hypophysitis (a condition that affects women in late pregnancy and postpartum, occurring in association with autoimmune thyroiditis and pernicious anaemia).
- Infection
- Trauma
- Pituitary surgery and radiotherapy.
- Kallmann's syndrome (isolated GnRH deficiency presenting with low LH and FSH, delayed puberty, tall stature, and anosmia. Some cases show a defective KAL gene on the X chromosome).

Acromegaly

Excess growth hormone (GH) production by a pituitary adenoma leads to acromegaly. In UK the annual incidence is 3-4 cases per million with a prevalence of 40 cases per million. Acromegaly may occur as part of the following syndromes:

- Wermer's syndrome or multiple endocrine neoplasia type 1 (pituitary, parathyroid and pancreatic tumours).
- Carney complex (spotty skin pigmentation, atrial myxomas, and endocrinopathies – Cushing's syndrome, acromegaly).
- McCune-Albright syndrome (polyostotic fibrous dysplasia, Café-au-lait skin pigmentation, endocrinopathies – acromegaly, Cushing's syndrome, thyrotoxic nodules).

The metabolic effects of growth hormone excess are mediated by insulin-like growth factor-1 (IGF-1) and include hypertension (40-50%), cardiomegaly, and diabetes (30%). Life expectancy is shortened by an average of 10 years due to the adverse cardiovascular effects of hypertension and diabetes. There is also an increased incidence of colonic polyps and colonic carcinoma. The diagnosis of acromegaly is suggested by elevated IGF-1 levels and confirmed by the failure to suppress GH to < 2 mU/l during a 75 gram oral glucose tolerance test.

The treatment of choice is a transphenoidal resection of the tumour, though bulky tumours with suprasellar extension may require a craniotomy. Radiotherapy works very slowly and is indicated if surgery is inadvisable, or if the excess GH production persists after surgery. Hypopituitarism develops in 50 per cent of patients within five years of radiotherapy and hence, these patients should be followed up regularly. The GH production can also be suppressed by somatostatin analogues such as Octreotide or Lanreotide, which are given subcutaneously or intramuscularly. The growth hormone receptor antagonist Pegvisomant is given subcutaneously and has been shown to normalise IGF-1 levels and improve insulin sensitivity.

LINKS TO BOOK ONE

1. Case 5, page 13. SIADH
2. Case 8, page 22. Primary hypothyroidism and polyglandular autoimmune syndromes
3. Case 27, page 77. Hypoglycaemia
4. Case 30, page 93. Sick euthyroid syndrome
5. Case 45, page 140. Acromegaly
6. Case 66, page 213. Pituitary incidentaloma
7. Case 83, page 281. Adult growth hormone deficiency.

Case 2

Hyperparathyroidism

A 59-year-old lady was admitted with a left Colle's fracture after falling at home. She had a previous fall six months ago and fractured the neck of the right humerus.

Na	145 mmol/l
K	3.9 mmol/l
Urea	6.9 mmol/l
Creatinine	120 µmol/l
HCO_3	16 mmol/l
Chloride	112 mmol/l

What is the diagnosis?

A. Hyperparathyroidism
B. Multiple bony metastasis
C. Osteoporosis
D. Multiple myeloma
E. Osteosarcoma

Answer (A)

DISCUSSION

Hyperparathyroidism

The combination of hyperchloraemia and metabolic acidosis suggests hyperparathyroidism. The following investigations are required:

- Serum calcium and phosphate
- Liver function tests including ALP
- Serum PTH levels

Hyperparathyroidism may occur sporadically at a rate of one case per 2,000 of the UK population. When hyperparathyroidism occurs in people below 40 years of age, one should look for evidence of Multiple Endocrine Neoplasia (MEN), which have an autosomal dominant inheritance.

Type 1 MEN (Wermer's syndrome) comprises of tumours from the parathyroid, endocrine pancreas (gastrinomas and insulinomas) and anterior pituitary (prolactinomas and somatotrophinomas). Other conditions described in Type 1 MEN include carcinoid, thyroid and adrenal adenomas, and cutaneous facial angiofibromas. Type 1 MEN is associated with a mutation of a tumour suppressor gene located on chromosome 11 (11q13).

Type 2(a) MEN (Sipple's syndrome) comprises of medullary thyroid carcinoma, phaeochromocytoma and hyperparathyroidism (parathyroid hyperplasia is commoner than adenoma). Type 2a MEN is due to mutations in the RET proto-oncogene located on chromosome 10.

Type 2(b) MEN refers to the combination of medullary thyroid carcinoma, phaeochromocytoma, multiple mucosal neuromas and marfanoid habitus. Prominent corneal nerves, which can be visualised with a slit lamp, occur in both forms of Type 2 MEN.

Parathyroidectomy

Most patients with primary hyperparathyroidism are asymptomatic. In one study* with a 10 year follow up, only 27 per cent of initially asymptomatic patients developed evidence of disease progression (defined as one or more new indications for parathyroidectomy). Therefore, the place of parathyroid surgery in asymptomatic patients requires careful consideration. The recommendations by the National Institute of Health (1991) are summarised below.

*Indications for surgery in asymptomatic cases of primary hyperparathyroidism***

- Serum calcium > 3.0 mmol/l
- Marked hypercalciuria: urine calcium > 10 mmol/day (or > 400 mg/day)
- Established complications: nephrolithiasis, osteitis fibrosa cystica
- Established osteoporosis (Tscore ≤ – 2.5)

- Reduction in creatinine clearance by > 30 per cent
- Age < 50 years

Other reasons for surgery may include: osteopenia, previous non-traumatic fractures, peri-menopause women, vitamin-D deficiency.

REFERENCES

* Silverberg SJ, et al. A 10-year prospective study of primary hyperparathyroidism with or without parathyroid surgery. N Eng J Med 1999;341:1249-55.

** National Institute of Health. Consensus development conference on the management of asymptomatic primary hyperparathyroidism. Journal of bone and mineral research 1991;6:s9-13.

LINKS TO BOOK ONE

1. Case 2, page 4. Hypocalcaemia
2. Case 21, page 58. Hypercalcaemia
3. Case 23, page 67. Osteoporosis
4. Case 49, page 149. Familial hypocalciuric hypercalcaemia
5. Case 62, page 197. Hypophosphataemic osteomalacia
6. Case 78, page 261. Osteomalacia and phenytoin
7. Case 84, page 285. Vitamin D deficiency and osteomalacia.

Case 3

Ectopic ACTH Syndrome

A 55-year-old lady was referred for investigation of backache. She also had weakness of the legs, generalised fatigue and two stones weight loss over the last three months. She was a heavy smoker, but without any significant past medical history. Her blood pressure was 168/94 mmHg.

Initial investigations were as follows:

Na	132 mmol/l
K	3.2 mmol/l
Urea	10 mmol/l
Creatinine	110 μmol/l
Glucose	8.2 mmol/l
ESR	110 mm/h
Hb	10.2 g/dl
WBC	8.4 x 10^9/l
Platelets	96 x 10^9/l
MCV	92 fl

Chest X- ray showed a right hilar mass

The medical registrar arranged the following investigations:

- Serum cortisol 09.00 hours 1,012 nmol/l
  24.00 hours 1,090 nmol/l
- Dexamethasone 2 mg qds was given for 48 hours and the repeat serum cortisol at 09.00 hours was 980 nmol/l.

What is the next most important investigation?

A. Bronchoscopy
B. High resolution CT scan of the chest
C. Glucose tolerance test

D. CRH test
E. ACTH levels

Answer (A)

DISCUSSION

Ectopic ACTH Syndrome

Possible causes for this patient's muscular weakness are hypercortisolaemia (i.e. Cushing's syndrome), hypokalaemia and paraneoplastic myopathy. Bronchoscopy and bronchial biopsy showed a bronchogenic carcinoma with ectopic ACTH secretion causing weight loss, hypokalaemia and hypertension. Cortisol has the same affinity as aldosterone for the mineralocorticoid receptor in the distal renal tubule and leads to retention of sodium, hypertension and hypokalaemia. The enzyme 11 β-hydroxysteroid dehydrogenase (11β-HSD) converts cortisol to cortisone and in doing so prevents the mineralocorticoid effects of cortisol being expressed. However, high levels of cortisol are able to overwhelm the 11β-HSD enzymes.

Tumours that produce ectopic ACTH secretion are small cell carcinoma of lung (the most common cause of ectopic ACTH syndrome – being responsible for 50% of cases), carcinoid tumours (lung, thymus, pancreas and gut), phaeochromocytoma and medullary thyroid carcinoma. The treatment is surgical removal of the primary tumour that is the ectopic source of ACTH production. If this is not possible, the remaining options are bilateral adrenalectomy (with provision of glucocorticoid and mineralocorticoid hormone replacement post-operatively), or suppression of adrenal cortisol production by medications such as metyrapone.

Diagnostic workup in Cushing's syndrome

Cushing's syndrome can be ACTH-dependent or ACTH-independent.

ACTH-dependent (80% of Cushing's syndrome)

- Pituitary adenoma (i.e. Cushing's disease)
- Ectopic ACTH
- Ectopic CRH
- ACTH use

ACTH-independent (20% of cases)

- Adrenal adenomas
- Adrenal carcinomas
- Adrenal nodular hyperplasia (including Carney complex)
- Corticosteroid use

In Cushing's syndrome, there is excessive cortisol production with loss of the normal circadian rhythm. For in-patients a midnight plasma cortisol above 50 nmol/l and an elevated urinary free cortisol (UFC) are useful markers of excessive cortisol secretion (normal range for UFC = 50-180 nmol/24h). The overnight dexamethasone suppression test is a useful screening test in out-patients: 1 mg of dexamethasone is given at midnight and plasma cortisol measured at 09.00 hours should be < 50 nmol/l in normal subjects.

The following investigations may elucidate the cause of Cushing's syndrome:

- ACTH levels at 09.00 hours (reference range 10-80 ng/l). Ectopic ACTH levels are generally very high (typically > 200 ng/l). In Cushing's disease ACTH levels could be normal, slightly elevated or high. In adrenal causes of Cushing's syndrome ACTH levels are usually low (< 10 ng/l) or undetectable.
- High dose dexamethasone test: 2 mg of dexamethasone is given 6 hourly for 48 hours. Urine and plasma cortisols should fall by 50 per cent. This response is expected in 80 per cent of patients with Cushing's disease and 20 per cent of patients with ectopic ACTH.
- Corticotrophin releasing hormone (CRH) test. In Cushing's disease, in response to 100 μg of CRH administered intravenously, levels of ACTH rise by 50 per cent, but there is no change in ectopic ACTH.
- The CRH test can be combined with measurement of the inferior petrosal vein ACTH, which is three times greater than peripheral vein ACTH in Cushing's disease. This is currently the best method for distinguishing between pituitary ACTH dependent Cushing's disease and ectopic ACTH syndrome.
- Diagnostic imaging methods include the following:
  - Pituitary CT or MRI if the above tests suggest pituitary adenoma (Cushing's disease)
  - Adrenal CT or MRI if an adrenal lesion is likely

- CT or MRI of the chest may detect small cell lung tumours that are responsible for ectopic ACTH production.
- Neuroendocrine tumours contain receptors for somatostatin. Octreotide is an analogue of somatostatin and ^{111}Indium labelled octreotide scans may detect those occult tumours that are missed by CT or MRI.

Pseudo-Cushing's syndrome

Patients with alcoholism and a primary diagnosis of depression may show features of pseudo-Cushing's syndrome, which is characterised by:

- Clinical features of Cushing's syndrome
- Excessive cortisol production including elevated plasma cortisol (with loss of diurnal rhythm) and elevated urinary free cortisol
- Resolution of cortisol excess on treatment of the underlying alcoholism or depression
- Abstaining from alcohol for five days will return the cortisol levels to normal
- Depression can occur as a secondary complication in patients with Cushing's syndrome and may cause diagnostic difficulty. A trial of antidepressants may be needed in any severely depressed patients with features of Cushing's syndrome. Successful anti-depressive treatment will restore normal cortisol levels in those with a primary diagnosis of depression.
- Depressed patients retain a normal rise in cortisol in response to insulin-induced hypoglycaemia, but this is absent in the majority of patients with Cushing's syndrome.

Cyclical Cushing's syndrome

This is characterised by:

- Unexplained cyclical or random variation in cortisol production.
- Improvement in symptoms and signs of Cushing's syndrome during periods of normal cortisol production.
- Spontaneous remission can occur which may last several years. Consequently, these patients require follow up and retesting for hypercortisolaemia.

Carney complex

This is a familial condition characterised by:

- Spotty skin pigmentation (lentigines on the face, lips and eyelids).
- Myxomas (especially atrial myxoma) and other soft tissue tumours, such as Schwannoma and breast adenoma.
- Endocrinopathies (Cushing's syndrome, acromegaly, thyroid adenoma, ovarian cysts).
- The most common endocrine disorder is Cushing's syndrome (seen in 30% of patients with Carney complex). The adrenal glands are stuttered with numerous black nodules < 6 mm in size and are visible on CT scan. This adrenal pathology is sometimes called primary pigmented nodular adrenocortical disease, or PPNAD.
- Mutation on chromosome 17 for Protein Kinase A regulatory subunit 1α (PRKARIA), which is a tumour suppressor gene.

Case 4

Nephrogenic Diabetes Insipidus

A 72-year-old man was referred to the medical out-patient clinic with a history of polyuria and polydipsia. He was not on any regular medications.

Urea	7.6 mmol/l
Glucose	5.6 mmol/l
Corrected calcium	2.46 mmol/l

A water deprivation test was performed during which desmopressin was given at 15.00 hours:

Time (hour)	*Plasma osmolality (mosmol/kg)*	*Urine osmolality (mosmol/kg)*
10.00	314	298
11.00	310	290
12.00	290	314
13.00	294	306
14.00	324	315
15.00	314	328
16.00	300	318
17.00	302	316

What is the diagnosis?

A. Type 2 diabetes mellitus
B. Cranial (central) diabetes insipidus
C. Psychogenic (primary) polydipsia
D. Syndrome of inappropriate ADH secretion
E. Nephrogenic diabetes insipidus

Answer (E)

DISCUSSION

Causes of polyuria and polydipsia

- Diabetes mellitus
- Diuretics
- Primary or psychogenic polydipsia
- Cranial diabetes insipidus
- Nephrogenic diabetes insipidus

Primary or psychogenic polydipsia

Compulsive water ingestion of more than 5 litres a day may lead to dilution of the extracellular fluid, suppression of vasopressin release and water diuresis. As a result, both plasma and urine osmolality are initially low, but urine osmolality rises above plasma osmolality during water deprivation.

Cranial diabetes insipidus

Failure to produce vasopressin seriously impedes water absorption from the collecting tubules in the renal medulla leading to diuresis. The urine osmolality rises in response to desmopressin (a vasopressin analogue). Causes of cranial diabetes insipidus include:

- Hypothalamic disorders
- Pituitary disorders
- Central nervous system infections
- Head injury

Nephrogenic diabetes insipidus

The renal tubules are resistant to vasopressin and urine osmolality does not rise in response to desmopressin. Causes include:

- Chronic hypokalaemia
- Hypercalcaemia
- Lithium
- Tetracycline
- Sickle cell disease
- Renal disease that damages renal medullary function, such as obstructive uropathy

Case 5

Addison's Disease (Primary Adrenal Insufficiency)

A 35-year-old Middle Eastern man was admitted to the medical ward with a 3 months history of diarrhoea, which occurred 5 to 7 times a day, but without blood loss. There was a 6 kg weight loss during this period. He was a heavy smoker. The chest and abdomen were unremarkable on examination.

Na	125 mmol/l
K	5.6 mmol/l
Chloride	94 mmol/l
HCO_3	14 mmol/l
Urea	18 mmol/l
Glucose	3.6 mmol/l
Corrected calcium	2.8 mmol/l

What is the cause of his hypercalcaemia?

A. Syndrome of inappropriate ADH secretion
B. Carcinoma lung
C. Addison's disease
D. Sarcoidosis
E. Thyrotoxicosis

Answer (C)

DISCUSSION

Addison's Disease

The diagnosis is Addison's disease or primary adrenal insufficiency. The manifestations of adrenal insufficiency are non-specific:

- Anorexia, nausea, vomiting, weight loss, abdominal pain, diarrhoea

- Increased skin pigmentation develop in areas exposed to the sun (face/neck) or pressure (elbows/knees); mucous membranes (inner surface of lips/inside mouth); scars that were acquired after the onset of the disease; and palmar creases in Caucasians. The pigmentation may be overlooked in dark skin individuals.
- Low blood pressure (lightheadedness)
- Tiredness
- Hypercalcaemia in Addison's disease could be due to dehydration (haemoconcentration and increased calcium binding to albumen), sodium depletion (encourages renal calcium reabsorption) and increased intestinal absorption.

Causes of primary adrenal insufficiency

The prevalence of Addison's disease in the UK is 39 per million and causes include:

- Autoimmune disease (80%), which may co-exist with polyglandular autoimmune syndromes type 1 and 2.
- Malignant destruction of the adrenal glands (the most common primary tumours are lung, breast, melanoma, hypernephroma, and lymphoma)
- Infectious diseases (tuberculosis, cytomegalovirus, fungal and HIV infections)
- Adrenal haemorrhage (Waterhouse-Friderichsen syndrome) occurs in meningococcal and pseudomonal septicaemia
- Adrenoleukodystrophy (Schilder's disease) is an X-linked condition in which defective β-oxidation of fatty acid by peroxisomes leads to adrenal failure and demyelination (blindness, dementia, and neuropathy). Affected males have elevated plasma levels of very-long-chain fatty acids.
- Infiltrative disorders (amyloidosis, haemochromatosis)
- Congenital adrenal hypoplasia is an X-linked disorder with mutations in a nuclear receptor called DAX-1. Adrenal failure in early life is followed by hypogonadotrophic hypogonadism.
- Congenital adrenal hyperplasia (21-hydroxylase deficiency and 11β-hydroxylase deficiency impair synthesis of glucocorticoids)
- Drugs that interfere with adrenal steroid production (rifampicin, ketoconazole, metyrapone, aminoglutethimide, trilostane, mitotane, etomidate)

Investigations

The essential tests are:

- Synacthen tests
- ACTH level
- X-rays of the chest and abdomen
- Adrenal autoantibodies

Short Synacthen Test

Blood samples are taken for cortisol before and 30 minutes after 250 µg of synacthen given IM or IV. The three criteria for a normal short synacthen test are:

- The baseline cortisol should be greater than 150 nmol/l
- The 30 minute cortisol should exceed 520 nmol/l
- The increment in cortisol should be more than 190 nmol/l

Note: Patients on hydrocortisone (cortisol) can be converted to dexamethasone before conducting a synacthen test.

Long Synacthen Test

Plasma cortisol is taken immediately before and 5 to 8 hours after 1 mg of synacthen given IM on each of the three consecutive days. Patients with secondary adrenal insufficiency due to ACTH deficiency (from chronic corticosteroid treatment or hypopituitarism) will show a step wise increase in plasma cortisol over the three days with peak values > 700 nmol/l.

ACTH levels

ACTH levels are measured at 09.00 hours (reference range is 10-80 ng/l). A high plasma ACTH of > 80 ng/l with low cortisol suggests Addison's disease (primary adrenal insufficiency). Normal or low ACTH suggests secondary adrenal insufficiency.

Adrenal autoantibodies and adrenal calcification

Adrenal autoantibodies may be present in about 90 per cent of autoimmune cases. These anti-adrenal antibodies are directed mainly against 21-hydroxylase, 17α-hydroxylase, and the cholesterol side chain cleavage enzyme. Adrenal calcification may be seen in tuberculous disease.

Treatment of primary adrenal insufficiency

- Glucocorticoid replacement
  - Hydrocortisone (cortisol) 20 mg each morning on awakening and 10 mg at 6 pm

    or
  - Hydrocortisone 10 mg on awakening, 5 mg at noon, and 5 mg 6 pm

    or
  - Prednisolone 5 mg on awakening and 2.5 mg at 6 pm

    or
  - Dexamethasone 0.75-1 mg on awakening

Note: Dexamethasone and prednisolone are longer acting, can be given once or twice a day, and may be more effective in suppressing pigmentation and ACTH levels.

- Mineralocorticoid replacement
  - Fludrocortisone 50-100 micrograms each morning.
- *Patient education:* They should increase the dose of glucocorticoid during illness and consult their physician if vomiting or severe nausea prevents the intake of corticosteroid medication.
- Medic-Alert bracelet with details of diagnosis should be worn. Patients should also carry a steroid card with up to date information on their medications.
- Provide a 4 mg ampoule of dexamethasone and injection equipment. Instruct patient and relatives in subcutaneous or IM injection of dexamethasone if glucocorticoids cannot be taken orally due to severe nausea or vomiting.
- Regular medical follow up to assess adequacy of steroid replacement therapy:
  - Weight gain (= too much glucocorticoid)
  - Skin pigmentation should disappear with adequate glucocorticoid replacement and normalising of ACTH levels
  - Postural drop in blood pressure and hyperkalaemia (= insufficient mineralocorticoid)
  - Hypertension and oedema (= mineralocorticoid excess)
  - ACTH and cortisol day curves may be needed:
    - Early morning ACTH should be < 100 ng/l
    - Urinary free cortisol < 250 nmol/day

— Plasma cortisol before the morning, lunch time and evening doses of hydrocortisone should be between 150 and 300 nmol/l.

Note: Cortisol day curves are only possible in patients taking hydrocortisone.

LINKS TO BOOK ONE

1. Case 8, page 22. Primary hypothyroidism and polyglandular autoimmune syndromes.

Case 6

Adrenocortical Failure As a Result of Long Term Corticosteroid Therapy

A 72-year-old woman was brought to the casualty department after being found drowsy by her neighbours. Two days ago she had presented to her General Practitioner with generalised aches and pains, and poor appetite. In the last 5 year, she had been taking prednisolone 7.5 mg od for polymyalgia rheumatica. On examination, she was rousable and the Glasgow coma scale was 12/15. She was apyrexial with no lymphadenopathy or organomegaly. The pulse rate was regular at 100 bpm. The blood pressure was 140/68 mmHg in the supine position and 100/50 mmHg on standing. There was a grade 3/6 ejection systolic murmur over the aortic area.

Hb	15.5 g/dl
WBC	10.2 x 10^9/l
Platelets	320 x 10^9/l
Na	120 mmol/l
K	5.1 mmol/l
Urea	9.0 mmol/l
Creatinine	135 μmol/l

What is the diagnosis?

A. Primary adrenocortical failure
B. Secondary adrenocortical failure
C. Primary hypothyroidism
D. Hypopituitarism
E. Syndrome of inappropriate ADH secretion

Answer (B)

DISCUSSION

Secondary Adrenocortical Failure in Chronic Glucocorticoid Therapy

The postural hypotension and hyponatraemia without diuretic use strongly suggests adrenocortical failure. The acute adrenocortical failure in this patient was precipitated by an infection. The most common cause of secondary adrenocortical insufficiency is exogenous corticosteroid therapy causing suppression of pituitary ACTH release and adrenal atrophy. Unlike primary adrenal insufficiency, *ACTH secretion is deficient and hyperpigmentation is therefore, absent.* Mineralocorticoid secretion is also normal.

Case 7

Klinefelter's Syndrome

A 28-year-old man was referred to the medical out-patient department for infertility. He has been married for three years and his wife has one child from a previous marriage. On examination, he has gynaecomastia, his total height was 1.74 metre, the lower body height measured from pubis to feet was 0.9 metre, and the arm span was 1.82 metre. A slit lamp examination showed no evidence of lens dislocation.

What is the likely cause of his infertility?

A. Hypopituitarism
B. Homocystinuria
C. Marfan's syndrome
D. Kallmann's syndrome
E. Klinefelter's syndrome

Answer (E)

DISCUSSION

Klinefelter's Syndrome

Individuals with Klinefelter's syndrome have at least one extra X chromosome. Classic Klinefelter's has a XXY karyotype and occurs in 0.1 per cent of male babies, but variants include XXXY, XXXXY, XXYY. Rarely individuals with a XXY/XY chromosomal mosaicism are fertile and show few classical signs. Physical signs include:

- Growth of the lower body is relatively greater than the trunk and upper limbs
- Small external genitalia and testes
- Gynaecomastia due to excess estradiol is seen in 50 per cent of patients

Glucose intolerance, hypothyroidism, breast cancer, varicose veins, and osteoporosis are much commoner. Intellectual impairment and anti-social behaviour have been described. Androgen replacement in the form of testosterone, 100 mg IM every month, may help restore diminished libido, alleviate impotence and prevent osteoporosis.

The essential diagnostic investigations are:

- Semen analysis (spermatogenesis is impossible from the fibrotic seminiferous tubules)
- Hormonal assays including serum gonadotrophins (elevated FSH and LH), testosterone (impaired production from Leydig cells), prolactin.
- Karyotype analysis

Causes of tall stature

1. Familial: this is the commonest cause.
2. Endocrine
   - Hypogonadism
   - Hyperthyroidism
   - Growth hormone excess (gigantism)
   - Lipodystrophic diabetes: Berardinelli-Seip syndrome is an autosomal recessive disorder that presents with complete loss of adipose tissue, macrosomia at birth, insulin resistance and diabetes.
   - Multiple Endocrine Neoplasia (MEN) type 2b (patients with MEN type 2b show Marfanoid features)
3. Chromosomal abnormalities
   - Klinefelter's syndrome
   - Supermale (47XYY)
   - Superfemale (47XXX)
4. Miscellaneous
   - Marfan's syndrome: autosomal dominant disorder with mutation in the fibrillin gene that presents with aortic aneurysm, valvular regurgitations, long fingers (arachnodactyly), increased arm span, high arch palate, pectus excavatum, superior lens dislocation.
   - Homocystinuria: autosomal recessive disorder with deficiency in cystathionine synthetase that presents with mental retardation, osteoporosis, inferior lens dislocation, venous and arterial thromboses.

- Sotos' syndrome: increased growth occurs only in the first two years of life and the final height is normal.
- Beckwith-Wiedemann syndrome is due to increased insulin-like growth factor-2 and babies with this condition present with omphalocele, macroglossia, hypoglycaemia, and show increased post-natal growth. Wilms' tumour may develop.

Case 8

Hypernatraemia due to Dehydration

An 85-year-old lady was found on the floor by her carers and examination showed a fracture of the right femoral neck. She has been a diet controlled type 2 diabetic for the last 4 years. She was confused on admission.

Na	156 mmol/l
K	4.3 mmol/l
Urea	12.9 mmol/l
Creatinine	158 µmol/l
Glucose	9.3 mmol/l

Arterial blood gases (on air):

pH	7.40
PaO_2	11.2 kPa
$PaCO_2$	5.6 kPa
HCO_3	28 mmol/l

What is the most likely cause for her confusion?

A. Diabetes insipidus
B. Diabetic ketoacidosis
C. Hypernatraemia due to dehydration
D. Primary hypothyroidism
E. Diabetic nephropathy

Answer (C)

DISCUSSION

Hypernatraemia due to Dehydration

The most likely cause of hypernatraemia in this patient is dehydration. The arterial blood gases do not show the metabolic acidosis that is typical in diabetic ketoacidosis. Established hyperosmolar non-ketotic pre-coma (HONK) is usually associated with much higher blood glucose levels (typically 50 mmol/l; range 20-150 mmol/l) and greater plasma osmolality (typically > 350 mosmol/kg).

Calculated plasma osmolality = 2 (Na + K) + urea + glucose

In this patient, the calculated plasma osmolality is about 340 mosmol/kg (reference values are 280-300), which is in keeping with loss of water. The most appropriate treatment is rehydration with IV 5 percent dextrose and IV insulin to control hyperglycaemia.

Case 9

Lag Storage Pattern

A 63-year-old teacher consulted his General Practitioner for excessive tiredness. His past medical history was unremarkable apart from gastric surgery for chronic duodenal ulceration 30 years ago. Urine examination showed 1+ glycosuria and no other abnormalities. The following tests were arranged:

Na	138 mmol/l
K	4.2 mmol/l
Urea	6.8 mmol/l
Creatinine	112 μmol/l
Hb	12 g/dl
WBC	7.2×10^9/l
Platelets	136×10^9/l
Cholesterol	4.6 mmol/l
LFTs	normal

He was referred to a medical out-patient clinic where the senior house office arranged a 75 gram glucose tolerance test (GTT). The results are shown below:

Time (minutes)	*Plasma glucose (mmol/l)*	*Urine glucose*
00	5.2	00
30	14.3	++
60	9.4	00
90	2.4	00
120	3.1	00

What is the most appropriate action?

A. Reassurance and discharge the patient from the clinic
B. Advise dietary measures for diabetes mellitus
C. Check thyroid function tests
D. Arrange CT abdomen to exclude pancreatic tumour
E. Tell the patient he has impaired glucose tolerance

Answer (C)

DISCUSSION

The GTT showed a lag storage pattern, which is associated with previous gastrectomy or thyrotoxicosis.

LINKS TO BOOK ONE

1. Case 44, page 138. Impaired fasting glucose.
2. Case 45, page 140. GTT in Acromegaly.

Case 10

Cushing's Syndrome (Adrenal Adenoma)

A 45-year-old woman presented with a history of backache, weakness of the legs and weight gain of 12 kg. Her blood pressure was 220/120 mm Hg. She also had purplish striae on the thighs, truncal obesity and increased facial hair.

Glucose	16 mmol/l
Na	140 mmol/l
K	3.2 mmol/l
Urea	7.8 mmol/l
Creatinine	128 µmol/l
UFC	1,280 nmol/24h (ref 50 – 180)
DHAS	0.6 µmol/l (ref 0.8 – 9.3)
ACTH	< 10 ng/l (ref 10 – 80)
Testosterone	< 0.6 nmol/l (ref < 3.0)

What is the most likely diagnosis?

A. Cushing's syndrome due to adrenal adenoma
B. Cushing's disease (pituitary adenoma)
C. Addison's disease
D. Ectopic ACTH secreting tumour
E. Conn's syndrome

Answer (A)

DISCUSSION

Cushing's syndrome due to an adrenal adenoma

In Cushing's syndrome due to an adrenal tumour, the ACTH level is low or undetectable and the high dose dexamethasone (2 mg qds for 2 days) will not suppress the elevated cortisol concentrations.

The DHAS levels are frequently below the reference range in adrenal adenoma and usually above the reference range with adrenal carcinoma. Diabetes mellitus is seen in 20 percent of patients with Cushing's syndrome and impaired glucose tolerance can be demonstrated in the remaining majority of patients (75%). Treatment of Cushing's syndrome due to an adrenal adenoma is either adrenalectomy, which is curative, or medical therapy to suppress hormone production such as mitotane, metyrapone, ketoconazole and aminoglutethimide.

Case 11

Hypocalcaemia and Secondary Hyperparathyroidism

A 62-year-old woman presented with low back pain and X-rays of the lumbar spine showed osteopenia.

Na	134 mmol/l
K	4.5 mmol/l
Urea	6.0 mmol/l
Creatinine	113 μmol/l
Glucose	4.5 mmol/l
Bilirubin	18 μmol/l
Total protein	72 g/l
Albumin	28 g/l
ALT	18 U/l
ALP	336 U/l
Hb	8.7 g/dl
WBC	7.2×10^9/l
Platelets	88×10^9/l
MCV	110 fl
MCH	24 pg
Red cell folate	220 nmol/l
Ferritin	30 μg/l
Corrected serum calcium	2.1 mmol/l
Serum PTH levels	18 pmol/l (ref 1.6 – 6.9)

25-hydroxy vitamin $D_3 < 13$ nmol/l (ref 20 - 110)

What is the next most appropriate diagnostic measure?

A. Isotope bone scan
B. Gastroscopy and duodenal biopsy
C. Dexa scan

D. Barium meal and follow through
E. D-Xylose test

Answer (B)

DISCUSSION

The patient has hypocalcaemia with secondary hyperparathyroidism. There is also macrocytic anaemia with low levels of serum ferritin and red cell folate. Two possible causes for low levels of 25-hydroxy vitamin D_3 are malnutrition and malabsorption.

LINKS TO BOOK ONE

1. Case 2, page 4. Hypocalcaemia
2. Case 21, page 58. Hypercalcaemia
3. Case 23, page 67. Osteoporosis
4. Case 49, page 149. Familial hypocalciuric hypercalcaemia
5. Case 62, page 197. Hypophosphataemic osteomalacia
6. Case 78, page 261. Osteomalacia and phenytoin
7. Case 84, page 285. Vitamin D deficiency and osteomalacia

Case 12

Subacute Thyroiditis

A 34-year-old woman presented with a 2 week history of a severe sore throat, which interfered with swallowing. She was previously healthy and not taking any regular medications. On examination, she was anxious looking with a mild tremor and sweaty hands. The blood pressure was 120/80 mmHg with a regular pulse rate of 110 bpm. The chest was clear. The thyroid gland was enlarged and mobile, but there was no evidence of tonsillitis, pharyngitis, or lymphadenopathy.

Hb	11.9 g/dl
WBC	$9.3 \times 10^9/l$
Platelets	$234 \times 10^9/l$
Free T4	88 pmol/l

A provisional diagnosis of subacute thyroiditis was made.

Which of the following investigation would confirm the diagnosis?

A. Thyroid ultrasound scan
B. Blood cultures
C. ASO titre
D. Throat swab for bacterial culture
E. Thyroid radioisotope scan

Answer (E)

DISCUSSION

De Quervain's thyroiditis

De Quervain's thyroiditis is an acute thyroiditis probably of viral origin with transient hyperthyroidism in the initial stages of the illness. It is commonly associated with systemic features of fever and a high ESR. Usually there is also pain in the neck and tenderness of the thyroid gland. The thyroid isotope scan shows suppression of uptake in the acute phase. After a few weeks, hypothyroidism may follow, which can be transient or permanent. Treatment is with aspirin, or short course of steroids for severe cases.

LINKS TO BOOK ONE

1. Case 8, page 22. Primary hypothyroidism and polyglandular autoimmune syndromes
2. Case 30, page 93. Sick euthyroid syndrome
3. Case 36, page 111. Amiodarone induced thyroid disease
4. Case 46, page 142. Levothyroxine non-compliance

Case 13

Conn's Syndrome

A 36-year-old woman was referred to the medical clinic for investigation of muscular weakness, cramps, numbness and tingling in her hands and feet. Hypertension was diagnosed 4 years ago after the birth of her last child. She was on bendroflumethiazide 2.5 mg od. She was a life long non-smoker and teetotal. On examination, she looked slim (BMI = 22), her pulse was 70 bpm, BP 150/100 mm Hg, and the optic fundi were normal. There was mild proximal weakness, but no other neurological signs, and the rest of the physical examination was normal.

Hb	13.2 g/dl
WBC	7.4 $\times 10^9$/l
Platelets	345 $\times 10^9$/l
Na	145 mmol/l
K	2.8 mmol/l
Urea	4.5 mmol/l
Creatinine	72 µmol/l
Glucose	5.6 mmol/l
ALP	78 U/l
AST	32 U/l
Corrected calcium	2.4 mmol/l
HCO_3	32 mmol/l
Urinalysis	normal
CXR	normal
ECG	sinus rhythm, no evidence of LVH

What is the most likely diagnosis?

A. Hypokalaemic periodic paralysis
B. White coat hypertension

C. Accelerated hypertension
D. Conn's syndrome
E. Bartter's syndrome

Answer (D)

DISCUSSION

Conn's Syndrome

The majority of hypertensive patients (90%) have essential hypertension in which there is no remediable cause. The remaining 10 per cent could have some form of secondary hypertension. Patients under the age of 40 years are more likely to have an underlying treatable cause for their hypertension. The most common form of secondary hypertension is primary hyperaldosteronism, which is present in approximately 1 to 2 per cent of the hypertensive population. Consider primary hyperaldosteronism in the following situations:

1. Resistant hypertension
2. Hypokalaemic hypertension
3. Hypertension in young people (< 40 years)
4. Familial Conn's syndrome

Note: One third of patients with primary hyperaldosteronism are initially normokalaemic

Primary hyperaldosteronism

Primary hyperaldosteronism refers to autonomous hypersecretion of aldosterone with suppression of renin. The two most common types are Conn's syndrome and bilateral adrenal hyperplasia (other listed types are much rarer):

1. Conn's syndrome (or Conn's adenoma, aldosteronoma)
   - First described by JW Conn in 1955.
   - Accounts for 50-60 per cent of cases of primary hyperaldosteronism.
   - Peak age of onset is 30-50 years. Female to male ratio = 2:1
   - Excess production of aldosterone by an adrenal adenoma.
   - Conn's adenoma functions autonomously and independently of the renin-angiotensin system.
   - Therefore, aldosterone levels do NOT rise on standing and often show a paradoxical fall.

2. Bilateral adrenal hyperplasia (or idiopathic hyperaldosteronism)
   - Accounts for 40 to 50 per cent of cases of primary hyperaldosteronism.
   - Peak age of onset is 6th decade. Male to female ratio = 4:1
   - Aldosterone secretion remains sensitive to postural changes in renin and angiotensin.
   - Therefore, aldosterone levels rise on standing.
3. Glucocorticoid remediable aldosteronism
   - Autosomal dominantly inherited condition
   - Chimeric gene on chromosome 8.
   - Chimeric gene has two components that have been spliced together: the aldosterone synthase gene and 11β-hydroxylase gene for cortisol synthesis.
   - Consequently, aldosterone is produced from both zona fasiculata and zona glomerulosa, and comes under ACTH control.
   - Therefore, suppression of ACTH by corticosteroids will also suppress aldosterone production.
4. Renin-responsive adrenal adenoma.
   - Similar to Conn's adenoma
   - But aldosterone production is sensitive to the renin-angiotensin system.
   - Therefore, aldosterone levels rise in response to standing.
5. Aldosterone producing adrenal carcinoma (rare)

Symptoms

Aldosterone increases distal tubular reabsorption of sodium and enhances the loss of potassium and hydrogen. The end result is hypokalaemia and alkalosis.

- Hypokalaemia may be associated with muscle weakness, fatigue, and cramps. Chronic hypokalaemia induces nephrogenic diabetes insipidus (and symptoms of polydipsia and polyuria).
- Alkalosis reduces ionised calcium. Hypocalcaemia can manifest as numbness, tingling, Chvostek's and Trousseau's signs, laryngeal spasms and convulsions.

Screening for primary hyperaldosteronism

Screening methods for primary hyperaldosteronism rely on changes in the aldosterone/renin ratio in response to stimulation by furosemide, upright posture, and captopril. In normal subjects, furosemide and upright posture stimulate the renin-angiotensin-aldosterone axis. In primary hyperaldosteronism, there is autonomous excess production of aldosterone and suppression of renin, which is not affected by furosemide or posture. Captopril inhibits the conversion of angiotensin I to angiotensin II, which in normal subjects leads to a fall in aldosterone production and a rise in renin. In primary hyperaldosteronism, captopril has no effect on aldosterone or renin.

The following screening methods are described in the literature, but unfortunately, there is no agreement on threshold values and methodology (some laboratories measure plasma renin activity and others prefer renin mass; some use SI units and others prefer metric units).

- Random aldosterone/renin ratio (ARR)
- ARR after frusemide and upright posture: ARR is measured after taking 40 mg of oral furosemide and 4 hours of upright posture.
- ARR after IV furosemide: ARR is measured at 0, 10, and 30 minutes after 40 mg of IV furosemide.
- Plasma aldosterone suppression after captopril: plasma aldosterone is measured 2 hours after a 25 mg oral dose of captopril.

Aldosterone/renin ratio (ARR) protocol

In our hospital, we use the following out-patient protocol in the screening for suspected primary hyperaldosteronism.

- The protocol is used in hypertensive patients with persistent hypokalaemia, or if there is inappropriate urinary loss of potassium (> 30 mmol/day)
- Before doing this test ensure the serum potassium is normal (> 3.5 mmol/l) and the patient is off anti-hypertensive medications although alpha-blockers are permitted (see next section for details).
- Ensure the patient is on an adequate intake of sodium (100-300 mmol/day) and potassium (50-100 mmol/day).
- Collect blood for aldosterone, renin and electrolytes after patient has rested quietly for 10 minutes. Aldosterone and renin samples are collected into lithium heparin tubes.

- Transport samples immediately to the laboratory: plasma for renin is stored at minus 20° Celsius and aldosterone at + 4°Celsius.
- In our laboratory a ratio of aldosterone (pmol/l) to renin (pmol/ml/hour) greater than 2,000 is highly suggestive of primary hyperaldosteronism.

Notes:

- *In SI units, aldosterone is measured in pmol/litre. In some laboratories renin values are quoted in ng/litre/second or ng/ml/hour.*
- *In SI units, a high ratio of aldosterone (pmol/litre) to renin (ng/ml/hour) is > 750*

Test protocol for confirming hyperaldosteronism

- Many anti-hypertensive drugs can affect levels of renin (e.g. ACE-I, ARB, diuretics, beta-blocker) and aldosterone (e.g. aldosterone antagonist such as spironolactone).
- If possible, stop anti-hypertensive medications 3 weeks beforehand (6 weeks for spironolactone).
- If necessary control blood pressure with alpha-blockers, such as doxazosin, as these drugs do not interfere with the renin-angiotensin axis.
- Ensure adequate salt loading with slow sodium (see below).
- Salt loading can worsen hypokalaemia and low serum potassium will also suppress aldosterone.
- Consequently correct severe hypokalaemia and ensure serum potassium is > 3.5 mmol/l before proceeding with the following protocol.
- Logistically it is best to admit these patients on a Friday for a weekend stay to allow careful supervision including salt loading tablets, a 24 hour urine collection, and remaining supine overnight prior to blood testing.

Day 1 (Friday): Prescribe slow sodium in an oral dose of 1200 mg tds for 3 days.

Day 3 (Sunday): Start a 24-hour urine collection for Na, K and aldosterone.
Patient to be remain recumbent overnight.

Day 4 (Monday): Take blood for supine renin, aldosterone, electrolytes and repeat these after 30 minutes of standing.

Interpretation

A urinary sodium of > 250 mmol/day suggests adequate salt loading. The following values suggest hyperaldosteronism:

- Urinary potassium of > 30 mmol/day especially in the presence of hypokalaemia
- Plasma renin < 1 pmol/ml/h
- Plasma aldosterone > 500 pmol/l
- Urinary aldosterone > 50 nmol/l
- Postural changes in renin and aldosterone levels may differentiate between Conn's adenoma and bilateral hyperplasia
- In general, Conn's adenoma have higher levels of aldosterone, which do not rise by more than 30 per cent on standing, and there is often a paradoxical fall (see Table 13.1).

Table 13.1: Postural changes in plasma renin and aldosterone levels

	Renin Supine	*Aldosterone Supine*	*Renin Upright*	*Aldosterone Upright*
Conn's adenoma	Low	High	No change	Falls
Bilateral adrenal hyperplasia	Low	High	Rise	Rise

Adrenal imaging

- CT or MRI scan
- Small tumours < 10 mm in diameter may be incidentalomas and require venous sampling to confirm aldosterone production. (*Note*: an incidentaloma refers to the incidental finding of a non-functioning adenoma; small adrenal incidentalomas are common.)
- Iodocholesterol scan is not widely available

Adrenal vein sampling

- Useful if CT scan results are equivocal, such as small tumour (< 5 mm) and bilateral abnormalities.
- Aldosterone and cortisol levels are measured from both adrenal veins and inferior vena cava during an ACTH infusion.
- Adrenal to IVC cortisol ratio of > 10 suggests correct placement of catheters.

- Right adrenal vein can be difficult to cannulate
- Aldosterone and cortisol ratio (A-C ratio) from each adrenal vein is calculated.
- High ratio is present on the side with a unilateral adenoma.

Treatment

- Conn's adenoma. Adrenalectomy may cure hypertension in 70 per cent of patients. Spironolactone is used pre-operatively to control blood pressure and correct hypokalaemia. Patients who are unfit for adrenal surgery, or where surgery has failed, can stay on spironolactone.
- Bilateral adrenal hyperplasia. Spironolactone (25-200 mg od) is effective in controlling blood pressure. Gynaecomastia may occur with higher doses of spironolactone, but this responds to tamoxifen 20 mg od for one month and can be repeated a couple of times each year. For patients who are intolerant of spironolactone, amiloride or triamterene are suitable alternatives. Eplerenone is a new mineralocorticoid antagonist and does not produce gynaecomastia.

Bartter's syndrome

- Rare renal tubular disorder with an incidence of 1 per million of the population.
- Presents before the age of 5 years with muscle weakness, tetany and seizures.
- Defective Na-K-2Cl transporter in the ascending loop of Henle
- Salt wasting and volume depletion stimulate the renin-angiotensin-aldosterone system.
- Aldosterone acting on the distal renal tubule increases sodium reabsorption and enhances the loss of potassium and hydrogen.
- Consequently, there is hypokalaemic alkalosis.
- Patients are *not* hypertensive.
- Renin and aldosterone levels are both high.
- Treatment consists of potassium supplements and ACE-I.

Periodic Paralysis

Periodic Paralysis (PP) is a group of muscle diseases that present as episodic muscle weakness. The PP may be primary or secondary.

Primary periodic paralysis

- Due to an inherited defect in ion channels in skeletal muscle.
- May co-exist with myotonia.
- Associated with changes in serum potassium during attacks of weakness.
- Muscle weakness may be local or generalised.
- Sodium ion channel defect: this is associated with hyperkalaemic PP in which weakness occurs after strenuous exercise or during fasting. The weakness responds to carbohydrate refeeding.
- Calcium ion channel defect: this is associated with hypokalaemic PP and the weakness usually occurs after strenuous exercise or after a high carbohydrate meal. The weakness responds to potassium supplements (oral or IV). Attacks can be prevented by potassium sparing diuretics, including acetazolamide, triamterene, and spironolactone.

Secondary periodic paralysis

- Thyrotoxic periodic paralysis
  - Occurs in adults aged 20-40 years.
  - 0.1 per cent of thyrotoxic patients in the Caucasian population (and 10% of thyrotoxic Chinese men).
  - Proximal muscle weakness is precipitated by carbohydrate intake and exercise.
  - Can involve respiratory or bulbar muscles.
  - Hypokalaemia during attacks of weakness.
  - Treatment of the thyrotoxicosis prevents recurrence.
- Muscle weakness in association with hypokalaemia due to: hyperaldosteronism, liquorice abuse, laxative abuse, diuretics, etc.

LINKS TO BOOK ONE

1. Case 2, page 4. Hypocalcaemia.
2. Case 64, page 204. Liquorice abuse.
3. Case 97, page 336. White coat hypertension.

Case 14

Lesch-Nyhan Syndrome

An 18-year-old man presented with sudden onset of pain in the right foot. He has had similar attacks since the age of 10 years. His General Practitioner prescribed colchicine 0.5 mg qds and allopurinol 100 mg tds. Blood samples were sent for uric acid. Three days later, he arrived in the A and E department with a fever, a painfully hot left knee, and by now, the right foot was more swollen. The medical registrar drew attention to this young man's obesity, mental retardation and ataxia. The following results became available:

Hb	12.1 g/dl
WBC	11.2×10^9/l
Platelets	132×10^9/l
Bilirubin	38 µmol/l
Na	148 mmol/l
K	5.2 mmol/l
Urea	11.0 mmol/ l
Creatinine	132 µmol/l
Glucose	6.8 mmol/l
CRP	112 mg/l
Uric acid	0.61 mmol/l
Aspirate from left knee	no bacteria; long needle shaped crystals with negative birefringence under polarised light with red filter

What is the likely diagnosis?

A. Gaucher's disease
B. Niemann-Pick disease

C. Lesch-Nyhan syndrome
D. Pyrophosphate arthropathy
E. Friedreich's ataxia

Answer (C)

DISCUSSION

Lesch-Nyhan syndrome

Lesch-Nyhan syndrome is a sex-linked recessive disorder resulting from deficiency of hypoxanthine phosphoribosyl transferase. The enzyme deficiency leads to excessive purine synthesis and thereby results in hyperuricaemia and gout.

Gout

Gout is mainly a disease of men (male to female ratio is 10:1). It is seldom seen in women before the menopause. Its appearance before puberty suggests an enzyme defect. Uric acid is the end product of purine breakdown and the last two steps in synthesis are: conversion of hypoxanthine to xanthine, and xanthine to uric acid. The enzyme xanthine oxidase catalyses these last two steps.

The level of the uric acid is higher in men than in women. Hyperuricaemia is diagnosed when the serum uric acid is more than two standard deviations (SD) above normal, which are 0.42 mmol/l in men and 0.36 mmol/l in women. Uric acid is completely filtered by the renal glomeruli and reabsorbed by the proximal tubules.

Secondary causes of hyperuricaemia

1. Increased production of uric acid
   a. Increased turn over of cells due to:
      - Myeloproliferative diseases such as polycythaemia vera
      - Lymphoproliferative disorders
      - Tumour lysis syndrome
      - Severe psoriasis
   b. Increased purine synthesis de novo such as:
      - Lesch-Nyhan syndrome (see above)
      - Phosphoribosyl-pyrophosphate synthetase overactivity
      - Glucose 6-phosphatase deficiency with glycogen storage disease
2. Impaired secretion of uric acid

- Drugs: diuretics, low dose aspirin
- Renal failure
- Hypertension
- Lead poisoning
- Primary hyperparathyroidism
- Hypothyroidism
- Excess alcohol
- Starvation

Clinical presentations of hyperuricaemia

- Acute gouty arthritis. This usually affects the first metatarsophalangeal joint with sudden pain and swelling associated with redness, raised temperature and tenderness. Other joints could be affected such as the knees, wrists, etc.
- Chronic polyarticular gout
- Chronic tophaceous gout characterized by the presence of white-yellow deposits around the joints and sometimes in the ear lobe and Achilles tendon. These gouty deposits may ulcerate through the skin. X- rays of the bones may show associated bony punched out lesions
- Crystal cellulitis similar to infective cellulitis may occur in very severe cases
- Urate kidney stones

Investigations for acute gouty arthritis

- High ESR
- Leucocyte count may be raised
- Urate level > 0.60 mmol/l, but levels may fall immediately after an acute attack
- Joint aspirate should always be sent for culture to exclude infection and confirmation of urate crystals, which are needle shaped and negatively birefringent under polarized light.

Treatment of acute gouty arthritis

NSAID's are effective in the acute phase. If they cannot be used, colchicine is a good option, but frequent doses produce sickness and diarrhoea. Small doses of colchicine, e.g. 0.5 mg taken two or three times daily is equally effective in the acute gout and much better tolerated. In severe attacks, either oral or local steroid injections could be used. Avoid allopurinol (xanthine oxidase inhibitor) in the first few weeks after acute gout. The dose of allopurinol should be reduced in renal impairment.

REFERENCE

1. Morris I, et al. Lesson of the week: Colchicine in acute gout. BMJ 2003;327: 1275-6.

Case 15

Lead Poisoning

A 50-year-old demolition worker was admitted with abdominal pain, vomiting and passing hard stools once every two to three days. He was treated for peptic ulcer disease in the past with omeprazole. He recently had been on holiday to India. On examination, he was pale with tenderness in the epigastrium. In the mouth, there was a blue line around the gums. Rectal examination was unremarkable.

Na	144 mmol/l
K	3.5 mmol/l
Urea	11 mmol/l
Creatinine	127 μmol/l
Glucose	6.0 mmol/l
LFT	normal
Amylase	150 U/l
Hb	8.2 g/dl
WBC	7.6 x 10^9/l
Platelets	238 x 10^9/l
Blood film	hypochromia, microcytosis, target cells, and basophilic stippling
CXR	normal; no free gas under the diaphragms
Abdominal X-ray	no distension of the bowel or fluid levels
Abdominal ultrasound	normal study
Gastroscopy	normal

What is the most appropriate diagnostic test?

A. Whole blood sample for lead

B. CT scan of the abdomen
C. Bone marrow aspirate
D. Mesenteric angiography
E. Barium meal and follow through

Answer (A)

DISCUSSION

The following clues suggest the diagnosis of lead poisoning:

1. Previous occupation as a demolition worker
2. Acute abdominal pain in the absence of a surgical condition such as perforated viscus or intestinal obstruction.
3. Blue line on the gums
4. Basophilic stippling on the blood film.

The clinical features of lead poisoning

- Anorexia, nausea and vomiting
- Abdominal pain and constipation
- Blue line around the gums
- Peripheral nerve lesions such as wrist or foot drop
- Lead encephalopathy (confusion, seizures)

How may lead poisoning occur?

- Occupational hazard: demolition workers, burning paint, scrap metal dealers, or smelting workers.
- Domestic poisoning such as accidental ingestion of fluid from car batteries, or chronic ingestion of water from lead pipes (nowadays they are non-existent in the Western world).

Findings on laboratory tests

- Anaemia with red cells showing basophilic stippling
- Bone X-rays may show dense lines at the metaphyseal ends ("lead lines")

Diagnosis and treatment

The diagnosis established by:

- Whole blood sample for lead: after absorption 90 per cent of lead is deposited in the bones and much of the remainder is deposited in the red blood cells. Whole blood lead level is < 1.0 mmol/l, but levels of 1.0 to 3.8 mmol/l may occur with occupational exposure. Lead levels above 3.8 mmol/l are usually toxic.

- Urinary porphyrin assays
- The abdominal pain is best relieved by sodium calcium edetate. The blood levels of lead can increase once the patient is started on calcium edetate, indicating clearance from the body.
- Definitive treatment is withdrawal from further environmental exposure and a chelating compound such as sodium calcium edetate (the drug of choice) with BAL (Dimercaprol).

Case 16

Turner's Syndrome

A 16-year-old girl was brought to the endocrine clinic by her mother. The mother was concerned about her daughter who had not started menstruating. The girl was intellectually normal, but of short stature with a webbed neck and cubitus valgus. The registrar arranged for a series of investigations and also referred her to the cardiologist.

What is the most likely diagnosis?

- A. Mucopolysaccharidosis
- B. Progeria
- C. Klinefelter's syndrome
- D. Turner's syndrome
- E. Hypothyroidism

Answer (D)

DISCUSSION

Main features of Turner's syndrome

Turner's syndrome affects 1 in 2,500 newborn females. The karyotype is 45, XO, but 40 per cent are mosaics such as 46,XX/45,XO karyotype.

- Short stocky build and stature
- Sexually immature with infantile external genitalia
- Primary amenorrhoea
- Facial changes including epicanthic folds, micrognathia, deformed or low set ears, and low posterior hair line
- Webbed neck (40%)
- Cubitus valgus
- Hands: swelling of the dorsum and short fourth metacarpal

bone
- Congenital heart disease such as coarctation of aorta
- Horseshoe kidneys
- Type 2 diabetes occurs in 60 per cent of adults with Turner's syndrome
- Hypothyroidism due to autoimmune thyroiditis is common
- Normal Intelligence Quotient

Differential diagnosis of short stature

The commonest causes
- Familial short stature (delayed growth)
- Systemic diseases such as malabsorption, renal or hepatic disease, cardiac failure, and chronic lung disease
- Starvation
- Emotional deprivation

Other causes

- Chromosomal abnormalities such as
  - Turner's syndrome (45, XO)
  - Down's syndrome (usually trisomy 21)
- Endocrine and metabolic disorders
  - Cushing's syndrome before closure of epiphysis
  - Hypopituitarism
  - Hypothyroidism
  - Rare metabolic diseases (e.g. mucopolysaccharidosis)
- Skeletal disorders such as
  - Achondroplasia
  - Osteogenesis imperfecta

Achondroplasia	*Osteogenesis imperfecta*
– Autosomal dominant	– Autosomal dominant
– Short limbs (upper arms and thighs more affected)	– Recurrent fractures
	– Blue sclera
– Normal sized spine but often kyphotic	– Otosclerosis
– Large head	– Hyperextensible joints
– Prominent forehead	– Bowing of the legs
– Depressed nasal bridge	– Pectus excavatum
– Normal sexual development	– Kyphoscoliosis
– Normal IQ	

Observations on the growth

After birth, growth continues rapidly in infancy, but slows down thereafter until there is a second growth spurt in puberty, which in girls occurs between the ages of 11 and 13 years and in boys between the ages of 13 and 15.

At birth, the ratio of the trunk to the limbs is 1.7:1. However, the legs grow more rapidly than the trunk and by the age of ten these segments become equal and remain unchanged unless for specific reasons.

Some important measurements to assess growth

1. Height: stand on a firm horizontal surface
2. Pubic symphysis to ground: this is to assess the length of the lower limbs in relation to the total height.
3. Arm span: this is a measure of the limb growth. The arms are fully stretched and the distance between the tips of the two middle fingers is measured. Normally the arm span and the height are equal.
4. Assessment of bone age. This is determined by X-rays of the wrist (on the non-dominant side) and comparing it with standardised charts (Tanner, Greulich, Pyle).

Sex hormones and growth

Although excess androgens and estrogens lead to an increase in skeletal growth, they also have an important role in *skeletal maturation*. Androgens and estrogens excess in early childhood lead to an increased height in comparison to children of similar age, but early fusion of epiphyseal cartilages ultimately produces short stature. Conversely, the lack of the sex hormones delays the fusion of epiphyseal cartilages and leads to tall stature.

Case 17

Necrobiosis Lipoidica

This 40-year-old man has been attending a specialist hospital clinic for the last 20 years. During a routine clinic visit, he drew attention to an area of skin discolouration on his left leg, which is shown below.

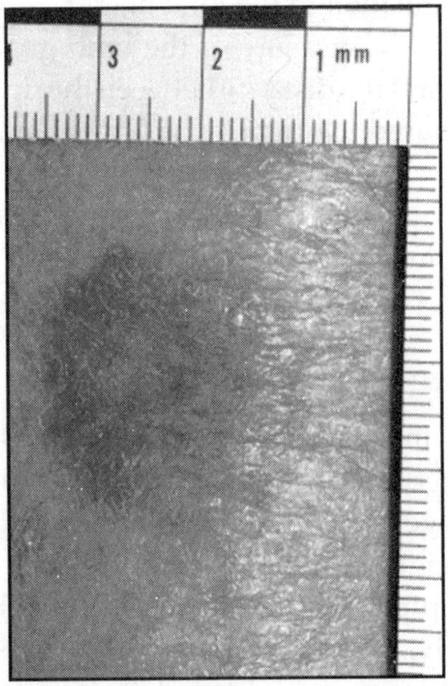

What is this lesion called?

A. Erythema nodosum
B. Necrobiosis lipoidica
C. Pseudoxanthoma elasticum
D. Acanthosis nigricans
E. Mycosis fungoides

Answer (B)

DISCUSSION

Necrobiosis lipoidica is characterised by a well-defined erythematous plaque with telangiectasia. The lesion is usually confined to the shin. Sometimes it will ulcerate and after healing, leaves a thin scar. It is commoner in females and usually starts in young or early middle life. About 50 per cent of the cases occur in non-diabetic individuals. The incidence of necrobiosis lipoidica in diabetic patients is around 0.3 per cent. The treatment is topical steroids under occlusion.

Erythema nodosum consists of tender purple-red nodular lesions occurring on front of shins. The lesions appear in crops over 3 weeks and fade away gradually to leave a bruised appearance. Ulceration and scarring is not a feature. Causes of erythema nodosum include the following:

- Streptococcal infections
- Tuberculosis
- Drugs such as contraceptive pills and sulfonamides
- Epstein Barr viral infection
- Inflammatory bowel disease (ulcerative colitis and Crohn's disease)
- Lymphomas
- Systemic fungal infections
- Leprosy

LINKS TO BOOK ONE

1. Case 55, page 169. Crohn's disease.

Case 18

Lipoatrophy

A 43-year-old woman was found unconscious at home and brought to the A and E department where general physical examination revealed the following abnormality on the right upper arm.

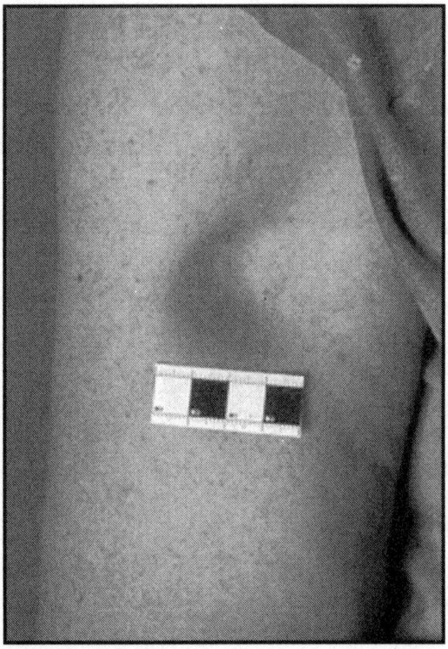

What is the most urgent investigation?

A. ECG
B. Blood gases
C. Blood sugar
D. CT brain scan
E. Chest X-ray

Answer C

DISCUSSION

Lipoatrophy

The patient was hypoglycaemic with a blood sugar of 1.8 mmol/l. The lesion on her upper arm is an area of lipoatrophy. It is due to a local allergic response to injections of animal insulin and can occur in both type 1 and type 2 diabetic patients. Affected individuals have high levels of anti-insulin antibody and lipoatrophic areas contain insulin and IgG immune complexes. These immune complexes induce the hyperproduction of tumour necrosis factor from macrophages, which in turn inhibits adipocyte differentiation. Lipoatrophy is rarely seen with human insulins and the newer designer insulins such as Lispro insulin.

Skin conditions associated with diabetes mellitus

- Bacterial skin infections such as boils and carbuncles
- Candidiasis
- Xanthomas
- Peripheral vascular disease and arterial ulcers
- Neuropathic ulcers
- Diabetic dermopathy: red brown flat topped papules
- Blistering on the hands and feet
- Diabetic stiff skin due to the glycosylation of soft tissues and the resulting changes in the physical properties of collagen. As a consequence, there is flexion deformity of the fingers, or cheiroarthropathy (see Figure 18.1), which should prompt a careful search for other diabetic microvascular complications, such as retinopathy.
- Diffuse granuloma annulare: these are characterized by small papules usually on the dorsal surface of the hands and feet. They are flesh coloured or slightly erythematous and asymptomatic. They are arranged to form a ring, or part of a ring. It may occur in the absence of diabetes mellitus.
- Acanthosis nigricans: these are areas of skin with a dark velvety appearance. The most common sites are the nape of the neck and axillae, and similar lesions can also occur at sites of continuous subcutaneous insulin therapy. Histologically there is hyperkeratosis, papillomatosis and increased melanin

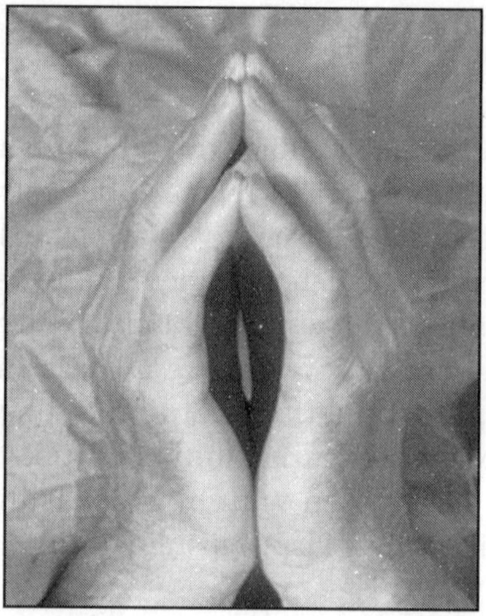

Figure 18.1: Diabetic cheiroarthropathy

pigment in the basal epidermis. Acanthosis nigricans is associated with insulin resistance and hyperinsulinaemia, and elevated insulin may have growth promoting effects.

LINKS TO BOOK ONE

1. Case 27, page 77. Hypoglycaemia.

Case 19

Plaque Psoriasis

This skin lesion was seen in a patient attending the rheumatology department with polyarthritis of the small joints of both hands.

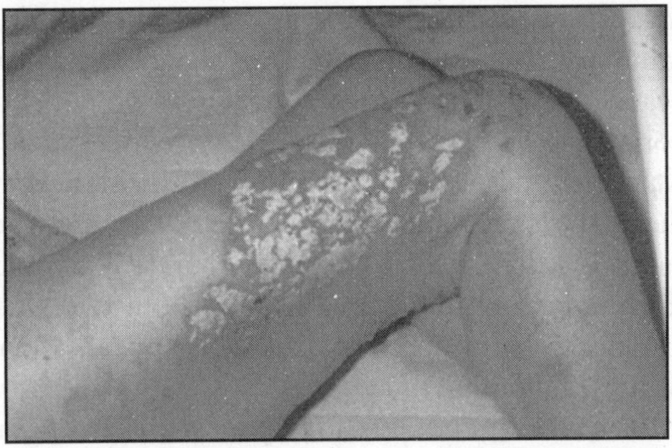

What is this skin lesion called?

A. Plaque psoriasis
B. Tinea corporis
C. Mycosis fungoides
D. Discoid eczema
E. Pompholyx

Answer (A)

DISCUSSION

Psoriasis

Psoriasis is a common skin disorder and affects two per cent of the UK population. It is characterized by well-demarcated, scaly plaques. Pathologically there is an increase in cellular turnover as indicated by acanthosis and parakeratosis. It affects males and females equally, but the age of onset has two peaks:

- Early 16 - 22 years
- Late 55 - 60 years

Clinical types of psoriasis

- *Chronic plaque psoriasis:* This is the commonest type and appears as scaly plaques particularly on the extensor surfaces such as the elbows and knees. It can affect the trunk. Koebner's phenomenon describes the appearance of new psoriatic lesions at sites of skin trauma. Normally the lesions are asymptomatic, but sometimes they may be pruritic or sore.
- *Flexural psoriasis:* affects the groin, natal cleft and sub-mammary regions. It is often mis-diagnosed as candidiasis, because the lesions in these "wet sites" do not show typical psoriatic scales.
- *Guttate psoriasis:* This is usually seen in children and young adults. The lesions appear as rain drop-like with an acute onset. The individual lesions are small rounded, or oval plaques, which appear on the trunk usually about two weeks after a streptococcal infection. The disease disappears spontaneously within 1-2 months.
- *Erythrodermic and pustular psoriasis:* The generalised erythrodermic form of psoriasis appears as wide spread pustules with malaise, fever, and possibly circulatory disturbance. The focal pustular variant affects the hands and feet, without systemic features.

Nail changes in psoriasis

Nail changes may precede the skin lesions in 50 per cent of psoriatic patients and take the following forms:

- Nail pitting
- Onycholysis (distal separation of the nail plate)
- Yellow brown discolouration
- Subungual hyperkeratosis
- Nail plate destruction

Arthritis in psoriasis

Psoriatic arthritis occurs in 5 per cent of the patients and may appear before the skin manifestations. There are the following types:

- Distal interphalangeal arthritis
- Peripheral arthritis (mono- or oligo-arthritis)
- Rheumatoid arthritis like lesions, but rheumatoid factor is negative.
- Spondylitis or sacroiliitis in those who are positive for the HLA - B27 antigen
- Arthritis mutilans: destruction and resorption of the affected bones

Case 20

Henoch-Schönlein Purpura

This elderly woman presented to her General Practitioner with abdominal pain, myalgia and the rash shown below. She also had a venous ulcer on the right leg that has been bandaged. Her General Practitioner did a urinalysis, which showed the following results:

Colour	light yellow
Glucose	negative
Ketones	negative
Blood	++
Leucocytes	+
Microscopy	presence of red cell casts

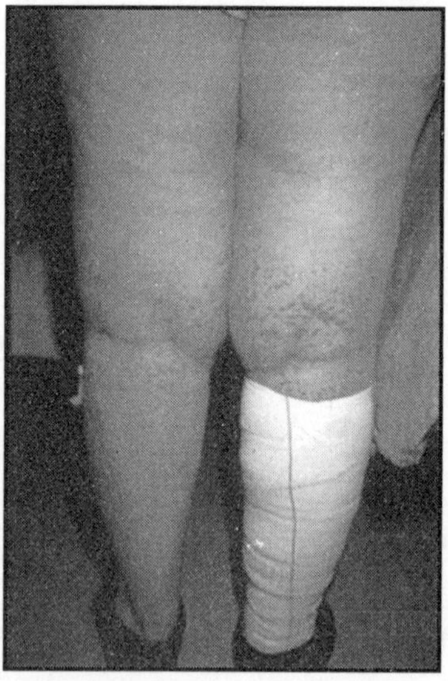

What is the likely cause of this rash?

A. Erythema nodosum
B. Erythema multiforme

C. Tinea corporis
D. Pityriasis versicolor
E. Henoch-Schönlein purpura

Answer (E)

DISCUSSION

Henoch-Schönlein Purpura

Henoch-Schönlein purpura (HSP) comprises of purpuric papular eruptions particularly on the extensor surfaces of the lower limbs, buttocks and trunk. It is a vasculitis that classically affects children particularly following an acute upper respiratory tract infection. About 25 per cent of cases of HSP occur in adults. Pathologically there is deposition of IgA immune complexes in the arterioles, capillaries, and venules. Clinically the patient may also have transient non-migratory polyarthritis, abdominal pain (bowel angina), and renal involvement (presenting as haematuria and proteinuria) may be seen in 50 per cent of the patients.

The American College of Rheumatology 1990 Criteria for Henoch-Schönlein Purpura

A patient is said to have Henoch-Schönlein purpura if at least 2 of these 4 criteria are present. (Note: the presence of any 2 or more criteria yields a sensitivity of 87.1% and a specificity of 87.7%):

- Palpable purpura: slightly raised "palpable" haemorrhagic skin lesions, not related to thrombocytopenia.
- Age at onset: 20 years or younger.
- Bowel angina: diffuse abdominal pain, worse after meals, or the diagnosis of bowel ischaemia, usually including bloody diarrhoea.
- Vessel wall granulocytes: histological changes showing granulocytes in the walls of arterioles or venules.

REFERENCE

1. Mills JA, et al. The American College of Rheumatology 1990 criteria for the classification of Henoch-Schönlein purpura. Arthritis Rheum 1990;33: 1114-21.

Case 21

Mycosis Fungoides

The patient is 60 years old and has had this itchy skin lesion for several years.

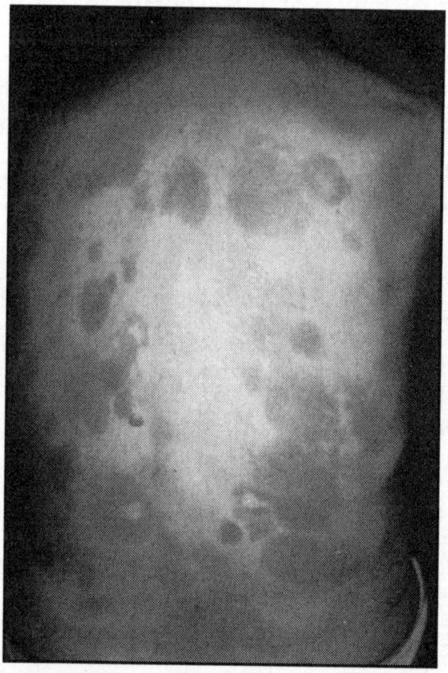

What is the likely diagnosis?

A. Tinea corporis
B. Mycosis fungoides
C. Discoid eczema
D. Erythema multiforme
E. Pityriasis versicolor

Answer (B)

DISCUSSION

Mycosis Fungoides

Mycosis fungoides is a cutaneous T-cell lymphoma, which appears insidiously as large erythematous patches and plaques, but could be eczematous or psoriasiform. Pruritis is common. The diagnosis is confirmed by skin biopsy. In most patients, the condition progresses very slowly over many decades. Treatments include topical steroids, locally applied cytotoxics, or PUVA. It may rarely progress as an erythrodermic variant with lymphadenopathy and peripheral blood disease, which is called the Sézary syndrome.

Case 22

Verruca Vulgaris

This patient presented with the skin lesion (shown below) to his General Practitioner.

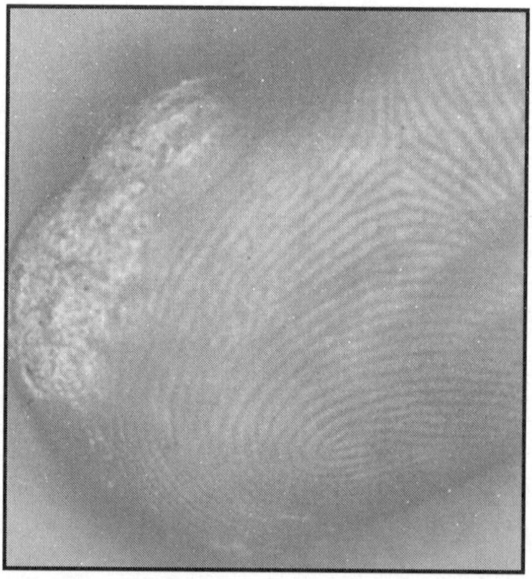

What is the likely diagnosis?

A. Verruca vulgaris
B. Malignant melanoma
C. Seborrheic warts
D. Warty epidermal naevus
E. Compound naevus

Answer (A)

DISCUSSION

Lesions of verruca vulgaris appearing on the hands are due to human papilloma virus infection. Discrete round papules with a rough surface are surrounded by hyperkeratosis. The same sorts of lesions on the feet are known as verruca plantaris. The lesions in seborrheic warts are multiple, skin coloured, or dark brown in colour and give a 'stuck-on' appearance on the skin. Warty epidermal naevus gives rise to brown linear plaque of warty skin. Compound naevus are rounded moles with a rounded or papillomatous surface.

Case 23

Scurvy

This 75-year-old elderly resident of a nursing home was admitted with anaemia and falls. He was cachexic and generally weak. He was not on any regular medications. His skin bruised easily and spontaneously (see photograph below). One month ago, he fell at his nursing home and attended the A and E department with a red swollen right knee. An acute haemarthrosis was diagnosed and he was discharged on oral flucloxacillin for one week.

On this admission investigations showed:

Na	146 mmol/l
K	4.8 mmol/l
Urea	2.5 mmol/l
Creatinine	122 µmol/l
Glucose	4.2 mmol/l
Total protein	45 g/l
Albumin	25 g/l
Bilirubin	16 µmol/l
AST	28 U/l
Bleeding time	7 minutes
PT	12 seconds
APTT	28 seconds
Anti-factor VIII antibodies	negative
Hb	7.9 g/dl
WBC	$6.2 \times 10^9/l$
Platelets	$346 \times 10^9/l$
MCV	87 fl
Ferritin	14 µg/l

Red cell folate	220 nmol/l
Vitamin B_{12}	180 pmol/l
Blood film	hypochromia and macrocytosis
Bone marrow examination	presence of megaloblasts, but no stainable iron
Vasculitic screen	normal

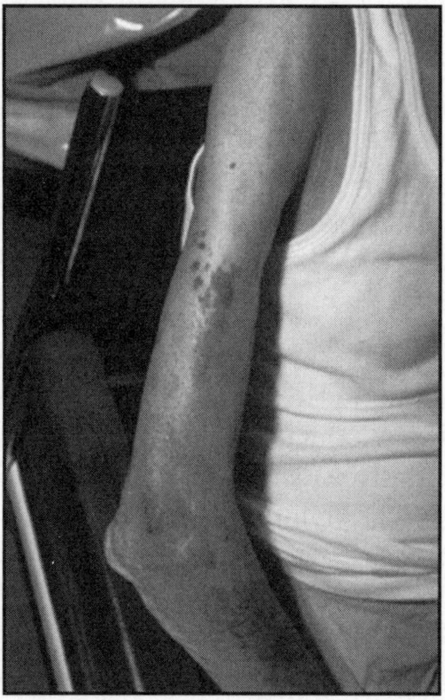

Malnutrition with hypoalbuminaemia and anaemia due to iron and folate deficiencies were diagnosed and further investigations showed:

• Faecal occult blood	negative
• Gastroscopy	small hiatus hernia; no ulceration or inflammation in the oesophagus, stomach and first part of the duodenum
• Duodenal biopsy	no evidence of coeliac disease

Permission for sigmoidoscopy and barium enema was not obtained. He was commenced on a high protein diet, oral iron and folate therapy. Three weeks later, his full blood count showed:

• Hb	10.2 g/dl
• WBC	7.2×10^9/l

- Platelets $480 \times 10^9/l$
- Reticulocytes 6 per cent

He continued to bruise easily and another fall in hospital resulted in a large haematoma in the right upper arm.

What is the likely cause of this skin appearance and the haemorrhagic tendency?

A. Thrombocytopenic purpura
B. Acquired haemophilia
C. Scurvy
D. Senile purpura
E. Henoch-Schönlein purpura

Answer (C)

DISCUSSION

The bleeding tendency was not due to thrombocytopenia or coagulation defects. Vascular purpura with bleeding tendency due to scurvy in an elderly patient with ascorbic acid deficiency is the most likely diagnosis. Malnutrition is the most likely underlying problem. Coeliac disease was excluded by normal duodenal biopsy.

Scurvy

Most animals can synthesize vitamin C (ascorbic acid) from glucose. However, this ability is not present in human beings and primates. Therefore, dietary deficiency leads to scurvy. The diagnosis of scurvy is usually clinical, but laboratory evidence of vitamin C deficiency can be documented by:

- Plasma ascorbic acid of < 11 μmol/l
- Low ascorbic acid concentration in the leucocyte-platelet layer (or "buffy coat") of centrifuged blood (normal range = 1.1- 2.8 pmol per 10^6 cells).

The main source of vitamin C is fresh fruits and vegetables. The reference nutrient intake for vitamin C is 40 mg a day and scurvy occurs when the daily intake is $\leq$ 10 mg. Vitamin C is essential for the hydroxylation of proline to hydroxyproline during the formation of collagen. This metabolic effect of Vitamin C deficiency accounts for most of the clinical features of scurvy, which are:

- Capillary fragility and haemorrhagic features
- Poor healing of wounds
- Bony abnormalities in children

The skin manifestations of scurvy

- Perifollicular hyperkeratosis (hair fragmented and buried in the skin)
- Peri-follicular haemorrhages
- Spontaneous bruising and ecchymosis
- Splinter haemorrhages in the nails

Other mainfestations of scurvy

- Bleeding into muscles and joints (atraumatic haemarthrosis)
- Swollen spongy gums: this occurs in people with dentition. The gums become swollen, with ulceration, bleeding and teeth loss.
- Ascorbic acid is involved in the regulation of iron absorption and distribution. Anaemia is due to malabsorption of iron or blood loss.

Treatment of scurvy

- High dose ascorbic acid: 250 mg od for a few weeks followed by 40 mg od.
- High intake of fresh fruits and vegetables.
- Left untreated scurvy may lead to confusion, hypotension, oedema, and death.

Case 24

Polymyalgia Rheumatica

A 75-year-old male normally fit and well and still involved in family business was referred with a two-week history of aches and pains. He has been unable to drive. His general practitioner tried simple analgesia without any help. In the OPD, he had aches and pains in the shoulders and thighs. He also gave a history of early morning stiffness. There was no muscular weakness or fever or weight loss. The investigations were as below:

Hb	10.2 g/dl
MCV	83 fl
WBC	9.8 x 10^9/l
Platelets	252 x 10^9/l
Bilirubin	18 μmol/l
AST	21 U/l
ALT	18 U/l
ALP	78 U/l
Albumin	41 g/l
ESR	118 mm/h
CPK	170 U/l
Urinalysis	normal
Electrocardiography	sinus rhythm
CXR	Normal

What is the most likely diagnosis?

A. Multiple myeloma
B. Metastatic bone disease
C. Viral polymyositis
D. Polymyalgia rheumatica
E. Fibromyalgia

Answer (D)

DISCUSSION

Polymyalgia rheumatica (PMR) is a disease of middle aged and elderly; it is rare before the age of 50. It affects both sexes but females are more often affected. The onset is often dramatic with the following symptoms:

- Pain and stiffness localized to proximal muscles (proximal myalgia); symptoms commonly start in the shoulder girdles and spread to the pelvic girdle muscles with striking symmetry.
- Morning stiffness with immobility severe on waking and persisting for hours.
- Associated common features include general malaise, fatigue, sweating, fever and depression
- Synovitis, particularly of the knee and wrist, and tenosynovitis leading to carpal tunnel syndrome can be seen.

Laboratory findings

The following tests are supportive for the clinical diagnosis:

1. Raised erythrocyte sedimentation rate/C-reactive protein is typical (A normal erythrocyte sedimentation rate may occur in 10 per cent of patients)
2. Normochromic normocytic anaemia is common
3. Elevated alkaline phosphatase, and γ-glutamyl transferase is common as an inflammatory reaction
4. No evidence of structural muscle damage; normal electromyographic studies and serum muscle enzyme values are normal

Diagnosis

Polymyalgia rheumatica (PMR) remains a clinical diagnosis suggested by evidence of inflammation and dramatic response to steroids.

Differential diagnosis of polymyalgia rheumatica

The main differential diagnoses are those disorders causing muscle aches (myalgia) and/ or stiffness, and bone pains including:

- Viral infections; any person having a flu in the past may remember the muscle pains
- Bacterial infections such as brucellosis

- Inflammatory polymyopathy and polymyositis (have raised CPK)
- Myopathies
- Rheumatoid arthritis can be of polymyalgic onset in elderly
- Connective tissue diseases
- Hypothyroidism
- Parkinsonism
- Bone disease such as metastasis, paget's disease and osteomalacia
- Malignancy including multiple myeloma

Treatment

Steroids are the treatment of choice with a starting dose of 10- 15 mg of prednisolone (orally) a day for the initial 4 weeks followed by gradual reduction of steroid treatment over 2 years minimizes the risk of relapse. The response can be monitored by ESR or CRP. Azathioprine may be added in some cases as a steroid-sparing agent after consulting the rheumatologist. Bone protection should be considered.

LINKS TO BOOK ONE

1. Case 23, page 67. Osteoporosis.

Case 25

Giant Cell Arteritis

A 71-year-old male presents with sudden onset pain in the right side of head for the last two weeks. He also had experienced pain in the right jaw forcing him to stop chewing his food for the past two weeks.

Hb	13.4 g/dl
WBC	9.2 x 10^9/l
Platelets	279 x 10^9/l
Na	134 mmol/l
K	5.2 mmol/l
Urea	8.2 mmol/ l
Creatinine	114 μmol/L
LFT	normal
ESR	110 mm/h
Electrocardiography	sinus rhythm
CXR	Normal

He was alert, mobile with no weakness or neck stiffness. His speech was normal. There was tenderness in the right temple. His heart rate was 98 bpm with a blood pressure at 184/98 mmHg. The fundoscopy was normal.

What is the most likely diagnosis?

A. Severe migraine
B. Acute maxillary sinusitis
C. Cerebral abscess
D. Benign intracranial hypertension
E. Giant cell arteritis

Answer (E)

DISCUSSION

Giant cell arteritis (temporal arteritis) is a systemic inflammatory vasculitis of unknown aetiology that affects medium and large-sized arteries. Almost any artery can be affected but the extracranial vertebral, superficial temporal, posterior ciliary and ophthalmic arteries are most commonly involved. The internal carotid, external carotid, and central retinal arteries are affected somewhat less frequently.

It usually affects patients older than 50 years and women are 2-4 times more likely to be affected than men. Its incidence is higher in Caucasians of European decent.

Clinical features

The onset is either abrupt or insidious. The symptoms are usually present for weeks or months before the diagnosis is established. A summary of the manifestations is given below:

Visual symptoms may be seen in up to 50 per cent of patients including;

- Sudden loss of vision commonly due to anterior ischemic optic neuropathy. This is an ominous sign and is almost always permanent.
- Blurring of vision
- Pain in the eye

Systemic manifestations may include fever, malaise, anorexia, myalgia, night sweat, and weight loss. These prodromal symptoms may occur for a few days or extend to weeks.

Headache is the main symptom of giant cell arteritis. It is usually localized to the temporal or occipital area and occasionally may be diffuse or bilateral.

Jaw claudication is a characteristic symptom.

Cerebrovascular complications occur in up to 25 per cent of patients including stroke, myopathy, peripheral neuropathy, and seizure.

Other rare presentations had been reported including aortic artery aneurysm, myocardial infarction, and visceral organ ischaemia.

The physical signs, which should be looked for include;

- Scalp tenderness especially over the temporal region often induced by very gentle pressure.
- Loss of pulsation and/ or tenderness and inflammation along the course of the temporal artery
- Bruits in the cranial or neck area.
- Optic disc oedema
- Visual field defects
- Central retinal artery occlusion
- Branch retinal artery occlusion
- Diplopia, ophthalmoplegia and nystagmus

There is a close relationship between temporal arteritis and polymyalgia rheumatica (PMR). Both conditions affect similar patient populations and frequently affect the same individual. Many think that these two diseases are actually different stages of a single disease spectrum.

Investigations

1. Temporal artery biopsy; should be done on the symptomatic side. When a lesion is obtained, it shows focal granulomatous arteritis with giant cells.
2. Elevated ESR or C- reactive protein (CRP) is usually present. If they are normal, the diagnosis is questionable. They are also used to monitor disease activity and response to treatment.
3. Normochromic normocytic anaemia is common with normal leucocyte counts
4. Alkaline phosphatase and serum aspartate aminotransferase may be elevated
5. Immunoglobulin levels may show polyclonal hypergammaglobulinaemia
6. Antinuclear antibodies and rheumatoid factor are negative

Treatment

High-dose corticosteroid therapy should be started, as there is impending danger of blindness in untreated patients. The goals of treatment are to reverse the disease and to prevent further progression. This is of utmost importance especially in the ophthalmic arteries to prevent blindness. Using constitutional symptoms, vascular symptoms, and the ESR findings as guides, the dose of steroids can be tapered off to a maintenance dose for at least 2 years.

LINKS TO BOOK ONE

1. Case 23, page 67. Osteoporosis.

Case 26

Bony Metastasis

An 86-year-old lady was referred to the rheumatology department with an 8 weeks history of low back pain. She had lost about 6 kg over the last 2 months. She had never smoked. She was cachectic on examination and liver margins were felt on abdominal palpation. There was spinal tenderness in the lumbar region. The isotope bone scan is shown below.

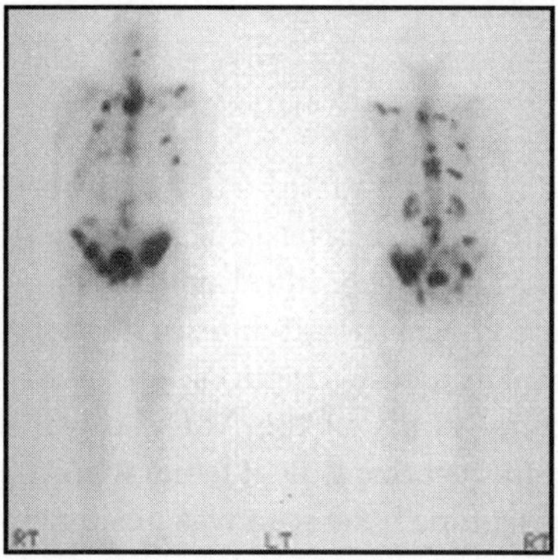

Hb	13.9 g/dl
Na	146 mmol/l
WBC	8.2×10^9/l
K	4.8 mmol/l
Platelet	340×10^9/l
Urea	8.0 mmol/l
Glucose	6.0 mmol/l
Creatinine	122 μmol/l
Bilirubin	16 μmol/l
Total protein	60 g/l

AST	28 U/l
Albumin	35 g/l
ALT	26 U/l
CPK	99 U/l
ALP	544 U/l
Corrected Calcium	2.9 mmol/l
Phosphate	1.9 mmol/l
ESR	120 mm/h

The raised alkaline phosphatase is possibly due to:

A. Hyperparathyroidism
B. Bony metastasis
C. Osteomalacia
D. Multiple myeloma
E. Osteoporosis

Answer (B)

DISCUSSION

This patient has a markedly raised ALP, which is originating either from the liver or the bones. The LFT's do not show evidence of hepatocyte necrosis. Hepatic infiltration by tumour (or granuloma) and cholestasis are clinical possibilities. The patient's presentation with bone pain makes a bony origin of the raised ALP much more likely. An isoenzyme study of the ALP can help to elucidate this problem. ALP from the bone is heat labile while that from the liver is heat stable. The isotope bone scan was positive in this patient and the chest X-ray showed a prominent right hilar shadow which proved to be an adenocarcinoma of the lung with both hepatic and bony metastasis. Useful investigations are:

1. Chest X-ray
2. Abdominal ultrasound
3. Skeletal survey or isotope bone scan
4. ALP isoenzymes
5. γ-GT or 5-nucleotidase

Raised ALP	
Bone disease	• Osteomalacia • Rickets • Metastatic carcinoma of bone • Paget's disease • Healing fracture • Hyperparathyroidism
Liver disease	• Hepatocellular jaundice • Obstructive jaundice • Hepatic metastasis • Primary biliary cirrhosis
Others	• Pregnancy (third trimester) • Temporal arteritis and other inflammatory conditions such as rheumatoid arthritis • Renal rickets (secondary hyperparathyroidism)

LINKS TO BOOK ONE

1. Case 65, page 206. Gallstone and fatty liver, interpreting liver function tests.

Case 27

Acute Gouty Arthritis

An elderly man was admitted with a painful knee joint. The knee was swollen, red, warm and tender with an effusion. His blood investigations revealed the following.

Hb	12.9 g/dl
Na	148 mmol/l
WBC	13.2×10^9/l
K	4.6 mmol/l
Platelet	440×10^9/l
Urea	13.4 mmol/l
ESR	50 mm/h
Creatinine	182 μmol/l
Glucose	6.0 mmol/l
Bilirubin	16 μmol/l
AST	28 U/l
ALT	26 U/l
ALP	80 U/l

Blood cultures were obtained and he was started on intravenous benzylpenicillin with flucloxacillin. A knee aspirate was sent for culture and sensitivity, biochemical assays, and examination for crystals. The latter showed needle shaped crystals, which were seen as negative birefringent under polarized light.

The picture of his hand is shown below.

What is the likely cause of his arthritis?

A. Septic arthritis
B. Acute rheumatoid arthritis
C. Pseudogout

D. Acute gouty arthritis
E. Pyrophosphate arthropathy

Answer (D)

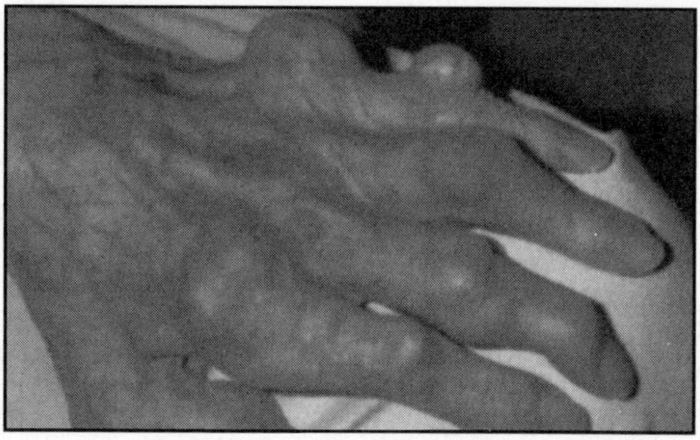

DISCUSSION

The causes of an acute red hot knee joint include:

- Septic arthritis
- Gonococcal arthritis
- Crystal arthritis: (gout and pseudogout)
- Trauma with haemarthrosis
- Haemophilia
- Occasionally: rheumatoid arthritis

Case 28

Churg—Strauss Syndrome

A 44-year-old lady attended A and E because of dry cough and breathlessness of 3 days duration. She denies fever or rigors. She was diagnosed to have asthma nine months ago. She had never smoked. In the past three months, she had been complaining of pain in the knees and right wrist. She returned from Thailand last year where she had worked as a teacher for ten years. Her general practitioner had arranged X-rays of the knees, wrists and hands, which were normal. She was on regular salbutamol inhalers and co-codamol as required. The oxygen saturation was 92 per cent on air. The blood pressure was 160/108 mmHg and the heart rate was regular at 104 bpm. She was not pyrexial and there was no lymphadenopathy or hepatomegaly. There were no signs of active arthritis in the knees, wrists, hands or ankles. The chest showed marked bilateral rhonchi. The CXR showed small patchy consolidation at the left lower zone. The electrocardiography shows a sinus tachycardia.

Hb	11.2 g/dl
Na	148 mmol/l
WBC	14×10^9/l
K	4.2 mmol/l
Platelet	244×10^9/l
Urea	10.2 mmol/l
Glucose	5.2 mmol/l
Creatinine	144 µmol/l
ESR	112 mm/h
Neutrophil	70 per cent
Lymphocyte	20 per cent
Eosinophil	10 per cent

The patient was admitted and started on oxygen, amoxycillin 500 mg tds and nebulised salbutamol (2.5 mg qds). Four days later her chest symptoms settled but she developed severe tingling sensation of the right arm with heaviness. Review by the medical registrar revealed that she had developed right wrist drop. Urine microscopy revealed granular and red cell casts.

What is the most likely diagnosis?

A. Allergic pulmonary aspergillosis
B. *Mycoplasma pneumonia* complicated by neuropathy
C. Systemic lupus erythematosus
D. Churg strauss syndrome
E. Tropical eosinophilia

Answer: (D)

DISCUSSION

The American College of Rheumatology 1990 criteria for the classification of Churg-Strauss syndrome (allergic granulomatosis and angiitis) is shown below:

1. Asthma
2. Eosinophilia >10 per cent
3. Neuropathy, mono or poly
4. Pulmonary infiltrates, non-fixed
5. Paranasal sinus abnormality
6. Extravascular eosinophils

For classification purposes, a patient shall be said to have Churg-Strauss syndrome if at least 4 of these 6 criteria are positive. The presence of any 4 or more of the 6 criteria yields a sensitivity of 85 per cent and a specificity of 99.7 per cent.

(Masi AT, Hunder GG, Lie JT, Michel BA, Bloch DA, Arend WP, Calabrese LH, Edworthy SM, Fauci AS, Leavitt RY, et al. University of Illinois College of Medicine, Peoria).

Skin lesions may appear including:

- Petechiae
- Purpura
- Nodules

The pulmonary lesions are transient, of variable size and could be unilateral or bilateral. The patient has raised inflammatory markers and the vasculitis can be p- ANCA positive. Usually they respond to steroids.

LINKS TO BOOK ONE

1. Case 33, page 103. Wegener's granulomatosis.
2. Case 39, page 121. Bronchial asthma.
3. Case 40, page 123. Obstructive lung disease.
4. Case 41, page 127. Restrictive lung disease.
5. Case 50, page 151. Amiodarone induced pulmonary toxicity.

Case 29

Polyarteritis Nodosa

A 52-year-old gentleman presented with symptoms of acute anteroseptal myocardial infarct. He arrived at the hospital within three hours and an electrocardiography showed ST elevation in V1-V4. He was treated with oxygen, intravenous fluids, diamorphine, oral aspirin 300 mg and tissue plasminogen activator. On the second day, he was haemodynamically stable with a blood pressure 118/68 mm Hg and heart rate 72 bpm. There were no features of cardiac failure. The diagnosis was further confirmed by a raised troponin T (6.6 ng/l) and raised CK (1500 IU/l). Initially the CRP was high at 110 mg/l with leucocytosis (15.2) and neutrophil at 80 per cent. On day 4, he developed right knee pain and swelling. On direct questioning, he had history of low-grade fever and polyarthritis affecting the knees and ankles. His general practitioner had treated him with NSAIDS and had been awaiting rheumatology opinion. The right knee was swollen and there was a livedo-reticularis rash over the shins, which had been missed on admission. The medical registrar reviewed the initial urine examination, which showed both blood and protein but the MSU had been negative in culture. The LFT's were also abnormal.

Bilirubin	12 μmol/l
AST	600 U/l
ALT	720 U/l
ALP	270 U/l
Total protein	80 g/l
Albumin	40 g/l

The registrar arranged other investigations.

Rheumatoid factor	Negative
ANA	Negative
ANCA	Negative

A provisional diagnosis of systemic vasculitis presenting as acute MI was made.

What is the most likely diagnosis?

A. Systemic lupus erythematosus
B. Churg-Strauss syndrome
C. Rheumatoid arthritis
D. Giant cell arteritis
E. Polyarteritis nodosa

Answer (E)

DISCUSSION

The patient has multisystem involvement presenting as acute MI but also had polyarthritis, livedo reticularis with abnormal LFT. The definitive diagnosis is made with one or both of the following:

1. Biopsy from the affected organ - the histology is seen as fibrinoid necrosis of the affected vessels with micro aneurysm formation, thrombosis and infarction.
2. Angiography showing micro aneurysms i.e. renal, mesenteric or hepatic vessels. The ANCA may be positive in 10 to 15 per cent of patients. Occasionally the condition may be associated with hepatitis B viraemia or antigenaemia.

Clinical manifestations of PAN

- Usually middle-aged man
- Systemic manifestations (fever, lethargy)
- Abdominal pain due to mesenteric ischaemia, ischaemic cholecystitis, pancreatitis
- Gastrointestinal bleeding
- Acute myocardial infarction or pericarditis
- Neurological (mononeuritis multiplex)
- Renal (haematuria, proteinuria, hypertension, renal failure)
- Dermatological (purpura, ecchymosis, subcutaneous nodules, livedo reticularis)
- Eye (chorioretinitis)
- Lungs - in classical PAN, lung involvement is rare.

Treatment

- Steroids
- Immuno suppressives as azathioprine

Follow-up of patient

Unfortunately, the patient had recurrence of acute MI involving lateral part of left ventricle. Eventually he had cardiac arrest and did not respond to cardiopulmonary resuscitation.

Table 29.1: Classification of vasculitis

Large vessel vasculitis	1. Giant cell arteritis
	2. Takayasu's arteritis
Medium vessel vasculitis	1. Polyarteritis nodosa
	2. Kawasaki disease
Small vessel vasculitis	1. Microscopic polyangiitis (ANCA +ve)
	2. Wegener's granulomatosis (ANCA +ve)
	3. Churg-Strauss syndrome (ANCA +ve)
	4. Henoch-Schönlein purpura
	5. Cutaneous lymphocytoclastic angiitis
	6. Essential cryoglobulinaemia

Vasculitis associated with other conditions

- Rheumatoid arthritis
- SLE
- Scleroderma
- Polymyositis/dermatomyositis
- Good Pasteur's syndrome
- Serum sickness
- Paraneoplastic
- Inflammatory bowel disease
- Infections such as hepatitis B, infective endocarditis, etc.
- Hypocomplementaemia.

LINKS TO BOOK ONE

1. Case 31, page 98. Cholesterol embolism syndrome – a condition that mimics vasculitis.
2. Case 33, page 103. Wegener's granulomatosis.

Case 30

Behçet's Syndrome

A 38-year-old Iranian immigrant attended the genitourinary clinic for recurrent genital and oral ulcerations for the past six months. He was married with two children (aged 10 and 12 years respectively). He denied any extramarital relationships. There was no history of urethral discharge. He had intermittent joint pains affecting the knee and ankles, which normally settled on ibuprofen obtained over the counter (without prescription).

At the clinic, it was also revealed that a local ophthalmologist had diagnosed right uveitis three months prior to this presentation. He was given local and systemic steroids with satisfactory response.

The right eye was slightly red. There were multiple aphthous like ulcerations, but without tonsillitis or cervical lymphadenopathy. There were few herpetiform lesions on the glans penis with no inguinal lymphadenopathy.

The medical registrar arranged FBC, CRP, U and E's, glucose, LFT, calcium and viral serology (including Herpes simplex). He also consented for HIV antibody test. After discussion with the consultant, the registrar made a needle prick over the flexor aspect of right forearm and asked him to come back two days later. On his re-visit to the clinic, a pustule had developed at the site of needle prick.

What is the likely diagnosis?

A. Reiter syndrome
B. Herpes simplex infection
C. Behçet's syndrome
D. Acute HIV infection
E. Secondary syphilis

Answer (C)

Discussion

Behçet's disease is a rare disease usually found in individuals from Turkey, Iran or Japan. However, it can be seen also in other countries including Europe and USA. Pathologically it is a systemic vasculitis of unknown cause. It is linked with HLA-B 51. The main features are recurrent oral ulceration (aphthous or herpetiform). To diagnose this disease, two of the following criteria are needed:

- Genital ulcers
- Eye lesions (anterior or posterior uveitis, retinal vascular lesions)
- Skin lesions such as erythema nodosum, pseudofolliculitis or papulopustular rash
- Positive pathery skin test (skin injury by a needle prick leading to papule or pustule within 24-48 hours).

However, other features may appear including

- Peripheral arthropathy (ankles, knees, elbows and wrists)
- CNS features including confusional states, meningitis and encephalitis
- Gastrointestinal features including abdominal pain, diarrhoea
- Renal or pulmonary involvement with vasculitic lesions

Neurological and ophthalmological complications require steroids and immunosuppressive therapy. Skin lesions and arthropathy may respond to colchicine.

Case 31

Rhabdomyolysis

A previously healthy 28-year-old engineer completed a 3-hour marathon for a local charity. Two days later he felt tired and suffered from aches and pains. His urine was dark brown in colour and reduced in volume. The pulse was a regular 100 bpm, blood pressure 158/102 mm Hg, and oxygen saturation on air was 96 per cent. He was clinically dehydrated. Urine dipstick analysis showed:

Urine dip stick	Specific gravity	1.018
	Blood	+++
	Protein	+++
	WBC	+++
Urine microscopy	No red blood cells	
	No red blood cell casts	

The medical registrar arranged for the following investigations:

Hb	10.1 g/dl
WBC	13×10^9/l
Platelets	340×10^9/l
Na	148 mmol/l
K	6.3 mmol/l
Urea	32.2 mmol/l
Creatinine	523 μmol/l
Glucose	6.8 mmol/l
CK	8,200 U/l

What is the most likely diagnosis?

A. Acute bilateral pyelonephritis
B. Acute interstitial nephritis
C. Pre-renal uraemia

D. Rhabdomyolysis
E. Lupus nephritis

Answer (D)

DISCUSSION

Causes of rhabdomyolysis include

- Trauma (e.g. fall, prolonged immobilisation, crush injury, vascular occlusion, burns, electrocution)
- Drugs (e.g. cocaine, opiates, ecstasy, amphetamines, statins)
- Hyperpyrexia
- Infection
- Myopathy

Laboratory features of rhabdomyolysis

- The serum creatinine (µmol/l) to urea (mmol/l) ratio is typically > 10.
- Creatine kinase > 2,000 U/l
- Hyperkalaemia, hyperphosphataemia, hypocalcaemia, hypomagnesaemia
- Myoglobinuria can appear as colourless urine, which is dipstick positive for blood, but no red cells are seen on microscopy.

Treatment

- Correct circulatory volume, oxygen saturation, and blood pressure
- Alkalinization of urine (pH > 6) with 1.4 per cent sodium bicarbonate to promote renal excretion of myoglobin
- Haemodialysis for severe hyperkalaemia

LINKS TO BOOK ONE

1. Case 29, page 91. Statin induced myositis.

Case 32

Renal Amyloidosis

A 78-year-old man presented with shortness of breath of 4 months duration, bilateral pitting ankle oedema and a dry cough. He had been attending a hospital clinic for a chronic medical condition over the last 25 years (his hand X-rays are shown below). About 30 years ago, he was treated with methysergide for a couple of years for migraine. His blood pressure was 190/110 mmHg. On auscultation, there was a fourth heart sound and bilateral basal crackles. Rectal examination showed a firm, diffusely enlarged prostate gland, which was not tender. He was started on diuretics, intravenous nitroglycerine and accepted for dialysis. He refused renal biopsy.

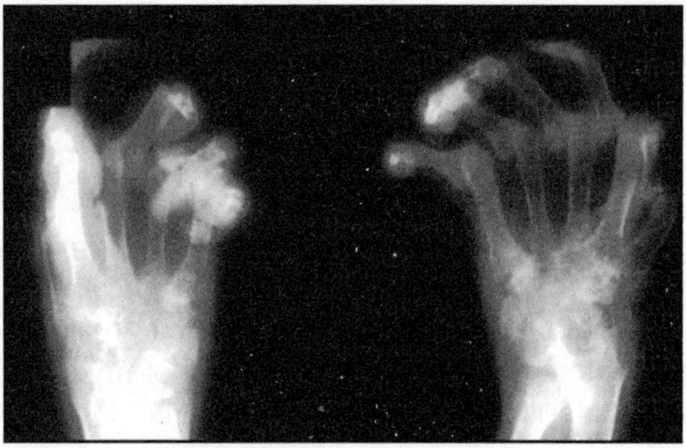

His other investigations were as follows:

Urinalysis	protein ++++
	red cells +
Na	129 mmol/l
K	4.3 mmol/l
Urea	31.0 mmol/l
Creatinine	630 µmol/l
Glucose	7.9 mmol/l

PSA	79 μg/l (ref <4.0)
CXR	Upper lobe diversion, heart size normal.
ECG	Sinus rhythm
ECHO	Mild left ventricular hypertrophy
Abdominal ultrasound	Right and left kidneys 10.2 cm and 10.7 cm respectively. No evidence of obstructive uropathy. There was mild enlargement of the liver and spleen; the inferior vena cava was patent.

What is the most likely cause of his renal impairment?

A. Renal amyloidosis
B. Retroperitoneal fibrosis
C. Benign prostatic hypertrophy
D. Renal vein thrombosis
E. NSAID induced nephropathy

Answer (A)

DISCUSSION

The X-ray of the hands shows severe bilateral deforming arthritis affecting the wrists, metacarpophalangeal joints, proximal and distal interphalangeal joints. These are compatible with chronic rheumatoid arthritis. The clues to the diagnosis of renal amyloid disease are:

- Long standing chronic inflammatory disease
- Normal sized kidneys
- Proteinuria
- The absence of obstructive uropathy on renal ultrasound

This patient is elderly and both hypertension and coronary artery disease are very common, which can account for the left ventricular hypertrophy and cardiac failure. Involvement of the myocardium with amyloid disease is rare in secondary amyloidosis.

Amyloidosis

Amyloidosis is a condition characterised by extracellular deposition of amyloid in the tissue and organs. The abnormal protein consists of ß-pleated sheets, which is insoluble and resistant to proteolytic enzymes.

Types of amyloidosis

I. *AL amyloid*

This is a form of plasma cell dyscrasia. An abnormal clone of plasma cells in the bone marrow produces immunoglobulins that are amyloidogenic. There is a clonal dominance of amyloid light chains (hence the name AL). It is often associated with:

- Myeloma
- Waldenström's macroglobulinaemia
- Non-Hodgkin's lymphoma

Clinically the condition may present as:

- Nephropathy and renal failure
- Cardiac failure
- Autonomic and peripheral neuropathy
- Carpal tunnel syndrome
- Macroglossia in 20 per cent
- Hepatomegaly

II. *AA amyloid*

This is due to deposition of serum amyloid A (SAA), which is an acute phase protein. The causes include:

- Chronic inflammatory disease (e.g. rheumatoid arthritis)
- Chronic infections (e.g. tuberculosis, bronchiectasis, osteomyelitis)
- Untreated Familial Mediterranean Fever

The common features are:

- Hepatomegaly and renal involvement
- Macroglossia does not occur
- Cardiac failure is rare

III. *Familial transthyretin associated amyloidosis*

This is an autosomal dominant hereditary condition.

Histological examination in amyloidosis

The common tissues used are rectal or gum biopsies. Amyloid appears as an amorphous homogenous substance that stains pink with haematoxylin and eosin, and stains red with Congo red. Under polarised light, it has a green fluorescence.

LINKS TO BOOK ONE

1. Case 61, page 194. Monoclonal gammopathy of unknown significance.

Case 33

Wegener's Granulomatosis

A 32-year-old man was admitted through the A and E department. He had been treated by the General Practitioner for a chest infection without improvement. His symptoms started 2 weeks ago with those of a common cold, including rhinorrhoea and dry cough for three days. He was advised to rest at home and take paracetamol as required. Three days later, he developed haemoptysis and right sided chest pain. He visited the General Practitioner again who gave him amoxicillin with regular paracetamol. On examination, he was apyrexial, not cyanosed or clubbed. The urinalysis revealed protein ++, blood ++, but was negative for glucose.

Hb	11.2 g/dl
Na	134 mmol/l
WBC	12.5×10^9/l
K	5.2 mmol/l
Platelets	275×10^9/l
Urea	10.2 mmol/l
Glucose	6.2 mmol/l
Creatinine	182 μmol/l
ESR	110 mm/h
Total protein	78 g/l
Albumin	30 g/l

ECG was normal. The chest X-ray showed two areas of patchy consolidation in the right lower zone. The oxygen saturation was 92 per cent on air. He was admitted to the medical ward. The blood gases on air revealed:

pH	7.38
PaO_2	10.1 kPa
$PaCO_2$	4.0 kPa
HCO_3	26 mmol/l

He was started on oxygen, IV antibiotics (flucloxacillin and cefuroxime in appropriate doses) and IV fluids. His condition did not improve. Review by the renal team suggested the following investigations: 24 hour urinary protein, MSU, renal ultrasound, vasculitic screen, coagulation studies, ASO titre, cryoglobulins, repeat chest X-ray, and renal biopsy. Three days later, the following results became available:

ESR	112 mm/h
CRP	120 mg/l
24 h urinary protein	1.5 g/day
Coagulation screen	normal
MSU	negative
Ultrasound scan	normal size kidneys with no evidence of obstruction
PR3-ANCA	65 U/ml (ref 0 – 6)
MPO-ANCA	15 U/ml (ref 0 – 6)

Anti-glomerular basement membrane antibodies were negative

Repeat CXR: The patchy consolidation in the right lower zone is larger with the development of cavitations.

What is the most likely diagnosis?

A. Tuberculous pneumonia
B. Wegener's granulomatosis
C. Renal carcinoma with pulmonary metastasis
D. Systemic lupus erythematosus
E. Goodpasture's syndrome

Answer (B)

DISCUSSION

Antineutrophilic cytoplasmic antibody (ANCA) is of two main types:

- Proteinase 3 (PR3) ANCA, which was previously called cytoplasmic ANCA (c-ANCA). This antibody produces granular cytoplasmic staining in neutrophil with indirect immunofluorescence assays.
- Myeloperoxidase (MPO) ANCA, which was formerly called perinuclear ANCA (p-ANCA). This antibody produces a perinuclear stain in neutrophil with indirect immunofluorescence assays.

In Wegener's granulomatosis, the PR3 ANCA is positive in 90 per cent of patients and the MPO ANCA may be positive in 10 per cent. The PR3 ANCA may be negative in Wegener's granulomatosis if the disease is limited to the upper respiratory tract. PR3 ANCA can be positive in microscopic polyarteritis. MPO ANCA may be positive in microscopic polyarteritis, Churg-Strauss syndrome, inflammatory bowel disease and rheumatoid arthritis without vasculitis. Wegener's granulomatosis and Churg-Strauss syndrome show a necrotizing granulomatosis, which is absent in microscopic polyarteritis.

Distribution of ANCA, eosinophilia in small vessel disease

	ANCA negative	PR3-ANCA (c-ANCA) positive	MPO-ANCA (p-ANCA) positive	Asthma and eosinophilia
Wegener's granulomatosis	~ 5%	~ 90%	~ 5-10%	Absent
Churg-Strauss syndrome	~ 30%	~ 10%	~ 60%	Present
Microscopic polyarteritis	~ 10%	~ 40%	~ 50%	Absent

LINKS TO BOOK ONE

1. Case 33, page 103. Wegener's granulomatosis.

Case 34

Hyperacute Graft Rejection

A 55-year-old diabetic with end-stage renal failure had a kidney transplant. Within 6 hours, there was almost complete loss of renal function and he passed only 20 ml of urine.

What is the most likely cause of his anuria?

A. Hyperacute graft rejection
B. Graft versus host reaction
C. Drug induced nephrotoxicity
D. Septicaemia
E. Acute graft rejection

Answer (A)

DISCUSSION

Hyperacute graft rejection is a humoral rejection caused by preformed antibodies in the recipient. These antibodies are produced by the following:

- Previous transplant
- Blood transfusions
- Pregnancy

The rejection occurs few minutes to a few hours after transplantation. T - lymphocytes are not involved in this type of rejection. Once the donor kidney is anatomised, the preformed antibodies activate the complement system leading to:

- Swelling and oedema of donor kidney
- Interstitial haemorrhage
- Thrombotic occlusion of the donor kidney vessels
- Renal infarction

The only treatment is removal of the transplanted kidney and restarting the patient on dialysis.

Case 35

Diabetic Nephropathy

A 54-year-old man has had type 2 diabetes mellitus for the past seven years. He has background retinopathy, microalbuminuria, hyperlipidaemia and exertional angina. He was attending the diabetic clinic regularly until one year ago when he defaulted. His General Practitioner has now referred him to the A and E department with symptoms of excessive tiredness, polyuria and lethargy. The current medications were metformin 500 mg tds, gliclazide 80 mg bd, simvastatin 40 mg od and atenolol 50 mg od. On examination, his pulse was regular at 72 bpm, temperature 36.6° Celsius, BP 180/120 mmHg, and BMI = 34 (weight = 98 kg). There was no evidence of cardiac failure, no carotid bruits and peripheral pulses were palpable.

Na	144 mmol/l
K	4.8 mmol/l
Urea	21.0 mmol/ l
Creatinine	270 µmol/l
Glucose	23.0 mmol/l

What is the most appropriate management?

A. Increase the dose of gliclazide to 160 mg bd
B. Add rosiglitazone
C. Hospitalise the patient to discontinue oral hypoglycaemic medications and initiate insulin
D. Rapid and effective lowering of blood pressure with sublingual nifedipine
E. Intravenous urography to assess renal function

Answer (C)

DISCUSSION

This patient has now developed severe renal failure and severe hypertension (BP 180/120 mm Hg). His diabetes is uncontrolled. The best therapeutic option is to admit the patient for:

- Arterial blood gases to assess his acid base disturbance
- Urinalysis (ketone, protein, blood), urine microscopy (casts), urine culture.
- IV insulin: stop metformin (unsafe in uraemia) and gliclazide (its metabolites are renally excreted and accumulate in renal failure).
- Assessment and correction of circulating volume; measurement of central venous pressure and urine volume.
- Blood pressure control.
- Review of diabetic complications: re-evaluate retinopathy; assess for foot ulcer risk.
- Renal team referral: renal ultrasound and 24-hour urine for proteinuria and creatinine clearance; education programme with decision on choice of renal replacement therapies (dialysis or renal transplant).
- Patient education (reason for clinic non-attendance; managing insulin therapy)

Choice of anti-hypertensive agent

Calcium channel blockers are good options for the treatment of hypertension in this patient, but sublingual nifedipine is contraindicated, as there are reports of stroke and heart attacks with this formulation. Therefore, oral nifedipine or amlodipine will be useful. An alternative is an alpha-blocker such as doxazosin. Both angiotensin converting enzyme inhibitors and angiotensin II receptor antagonists are probably unsafe at this stage. Intravenous nitrate can provide a controlled reduction of blood pressure and has a short half-life.

The recommended target blood pressure in people with diabetes is 130/80 mmHg or less (British Hypertension Society guidelines 2004). If ambulatory blood pressure readings are taken, the target value in mean daytime blood pressure should be 10/5 mm Hg less than clinic readings. The target blood pressures for diabetic patients with more than one gram of proteinuria a day should be less than 125/75 mm Hg.

Creatinine clearance

Creatinine clearance is one method of measuring glomerular filtration rate and requires a 24-hour collection and blood sample. In patients with stable renal function, i.e. where the urea and creatinine are not rising rapidly, the Cockcroft-Gault equation (Cockcroft DW and Gault MH. Nephron 1976;16:31-41) can be used for estimating creatinine clearance:

$$\text{Creatinine clearance (Cr Cl)} = \frac{1.2 \times (140 - \text{age}) \times \text{body weight in kg}}{\text{Serum creatinine}}$$

$$\text{For this patient, Cr Cl} = \frac{1.2 \times (140 - 54) \times 98}{270} = 37.2 \text{ ml/min}$$

Diabetic renal disease

In the Western World, diabetic renal disease is the most common cause of end stage renal failure. In the UK, approximately 1,000 diabetic individuals develop end stage renal failure each year. The majority will be patients with type 2 diabetes as this is numerically the more common than type 1 diabetes. About one third of patients with type 1 diabetes and a similar proportion of type 2 diabetics will eventually develop diabetic nephropathy. However, not every type 2 diabetic patient with proteinuria will turn out to have diabetic renal disease: in one quarter of these patients, the proteinuria is due to other pathologies (e.g. glomerulonephritis, renovascular disease). The presence of other diabetic microvascular complications, such as retinopathy and neuropathy, suggest the proteinuria is more likely to be diabetic renal disease, because microvascular complications tend to co-exist. A renal biopsy may be needed to clarify the underlying pathology. The main cause of death in type 2 diabetics with renal disease is coronary heart disease: about 75 percent of diabetic renal patients will die from it. In addition, there is a serious burden in peripheral artery disease and its complications (ulceration, sepsis, gangrene, and amputation). Therefore, other vascular risks such as smoking and hyperlipidaemia will need to be tackled aggressively.

The stages in diabetic renal disease

In the UKPDS, 11.4 per cent of patients with newly diagnosed type 2 diabetes already have proteinuria (defined as urine albumin > 50 mg/l). Each year about 2 per cent of diabetic patients undergo transition from normoalbuminuria to microalbuminuria; 2 per cent from microalbuminuria to macroalbuminuria; and 2 per cent from macroalbuminuria to end stage renal failure (UKPDS -64. Kidney Int 2003;63:225-32).

Stage 1 Normo-albuminuria phase

Hyperfiltration is mediated by an increase in nitric oxide production. The glomerular filtration rate is elevated and there is an increase in kidney size. It is postulated that increased hyperfiltration may cause structural damage to the renal glomeruli.

Stage 2 Micro-albuminuria phase

Microalbuminuria (20-200 µg/min or 30–300 mg/day) cannot be detected using the commonly deployed urine test strips in the clinic (hence the term *dipstick negative proteinuria*). Test strips specifically able to detect microalbuminuria are available such as Micral-Test, but false positives are common.

Early morning urine (EMU) i.e. the first aliquot of urine produced after recumbency overnight can be tested for microalbuminuria. Three EMUs are sent for measurement of the albumin (mg) to creatinine ratio (mmol) (ACR). Patients should refrain from heavy physical activity and sexual intercourse for 3 days before this urine collection. It is recommended that all type 2 diabetics should have annual screening for microalbuminuria. In type 1 diabetes, microalbuminuria screening should be done annually after puberty, or annually after 5 years of diagnosis. An ACR > 2.5 mg/mmol in men (or > 3.5 mg/mmol in women) indicates microalbuminuria.

As the degree of albumin excretion increases towards the high end of the microalbuminuric range, there is a fall in creatinine clearance by about 10 ml per minute per annum and an inevitable rise in blood pressure. Tight blood pressure control with ACE-inhibitors reduces the progression of diabetic renal disease with a 50 per cent reduction in the risk of progression from microalbuminuria to macroalbuminuria. Some evidence also exists for the beneficial effect of cholesterol reduction in preserving renal function.

In the DCCT study tight glycaemic control in type 1 diabetes reduces the chances of developing microalbuminuria by 34 percent. In the UKPDS study of type 2 diabetes tight glycaemic control reduces microvascular complications: a 1 per cent reduction in HbA1c reduced microvascular complications by 37 per cent (UKPDS-35. BMJ 2000;321:405-12).

Stage 3 Macro-albuminuria phase

Macroalbuminuria (urine albumin > 300 mg per day or > 200 μg per minute): *dip stick positive proteinuria.* Unfortunately, by this stage there has already been significant loss of renal function. Once macroalbuminuria has developed there is on average only another 5 years before end stage renal failure ensues. It is generally believed that once macroalbuminuria has developed tight glycaemic control will not delay the inevitable decline in renal function. Two trials have shown that the combination of angiotensin II receptor antagonist and ACE-inhibitor given for 2-3 years may reduce the decline in GFR by 15 per cent and study end points (doubling in serum creatinine, end-stage renal failure and death) by 20-25 percent. (RENAAL study, Brenner BM et al. NEJM 2001: 345:861-69 and IDNT study, Lewis EJ et al. NEJM 2001;345:851-60). The entry criteria for these two trials were type 2 diabetics with serum creatinine < 265 μmol/l and proteinuria > 500–900 mg a day.

Stage 4 End stage renal disease

The decline in creatinine is linear if the inverse creatinine (1/creatinine) is plotted against time. This allows an estimation of the time to reach end stage renal failure (arbitrarily defined as a serum creatinine of > 250 μmol/l). Referral to the renal team is suggested when the serum creatinine is > 150 μmol/l. (Management of type 2 diabetes - renal disease prevention and early management, NICE Guideline 2002; www.nice.org.uk). Decisions on either dialysis or transplant should be taken before the serum creatinine rises above 250 μmol/l.

The annual cost of maintaining a patient with end stage renal failure on peritoneal dialysis is £20,000 (or £34,500 p.a. for haemodialysis). The cost of a kidney transplant is £20,000 per patient with an annual recurring cost of £6,500 for immunosuppressive medication (figures from UK Transplant 2003, which is a Special Health Authority within the NHS, www.uktransplant.org.uk).

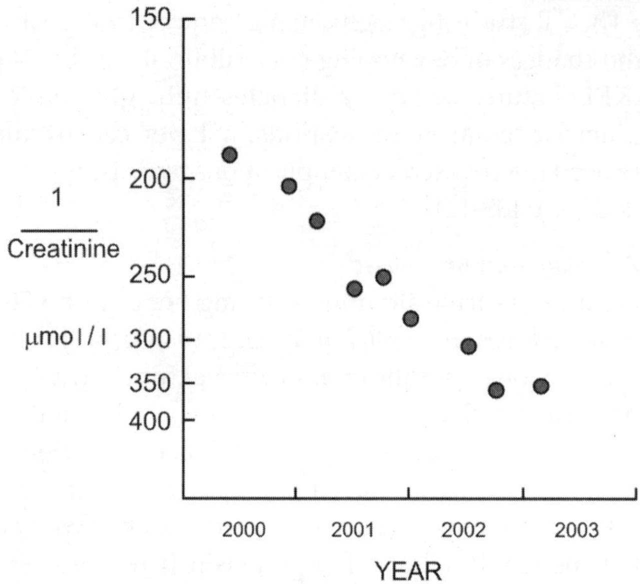

Fig. 35.1: The reciprocal of serum creatinine (1/creatinine) plotting against time (years) shows a linear relationship.

Table 35.1: Stages in diabetic renal disease

	Urine albumin	*GFR*	*BP*
Stage 1 Normo-albuminuria	< 20 μg per min	Normal or high	Normal
Stage 2 Micro-albuminuria	20-200 μg per min	Normal or high	Rising
Stage 3 Macro-albuminuria	> 200 μg per min	Falling	High
Stage 4 End stage disease	> 200 μg per min	Low	High

Notes:

300 mg of albuminuria = 500 mg of proteinuria
20-200 μg per min = 30-300 mg/day

LINKS WITH BOOK ONE

1. Case 32, page 101. Radiocontrast nephrotoxicity.
2. Case 44, page 138. Impaired fasting glucose.
3. Case 58, page 181. Familial hypercholesterolaemia.
4. Case 94, page 324. Ambulatory blood pressure profile: non-dipper.
5. Case 97, page 336. White coat hypertension.

REFERENCE

1. British Hypertension Society guidelines for hypertension management 2004 (BHS-IV): summary. BMJ 2004;328:634-40.

Case 36

Metabolic Acidosis with Normal Anion Gap and Ureterosigmoidostomy

A 76-year-old man presented with shortness of breath of two weeks duration. Forty-three years ago, he underwent left nephrectomy for renal tuberculosis and 16 years later underwent another abdominal operation. On examination, he was pigmented and hyperventilating.

Na	140 mmol/l
K	3.0 mmol/l
Urea	13 mmol/l
Creatinine	157 µmol/l
Glucose	6.2 mmol/l
Chloride	114 mmol/l

Arterial blood gases (on air):

pH	7.2
PaO_2	12.7 kPa
$PaCO_2$	3.3 kPa
HCO_3	15 mmol/l

What do these tests show?

A. Uncompensated respiratory acidosis
B. Metabolic acidosis due to renal failure
C. Metabolic and respiratory acidosis
D. Unsuspected salicylate poisoning
E. Metabolic acidosis with normal anion gap

Answer (E)

DISCUSSION

Metabolic acidosis with normal anion gap

This patient has a metabolic acidosis and hypokalaemia with a

normal anion gap. The latter is calculated as follows:
{Na + K} - {HCO_3 + Cl} = 12-16

Metabolic acidosis with normal anion gap can occur with the following:

- Renal tubular acidosis
- Ureterosigmoidostomy
- Severe diarrhoea
- Acetazolamide therapy

In ureterosigmoidostomy, the chloride is reabsorbed in exchange for HCO_3 and potassium.

Complications of Ureterosigmoidostomy

- Ureter stricture at the site of the anastomosis
- Reflux of the bowel contents into the ureters with consequent repeated pyelonephritis and chronic renal failure
- Ureteral neoplasm at the site of the anastomosis (which presents as rectal bleeding)
- Diarrhoea due to irritation of the colon by urine
- Hypokalaemia
- Hyperchloraemic acidosis
- Chronic acidosis leading to nephrocalcinosis and osteomalacia

LINKS TO BOOK ONE

1. Case 47, page 144. Chronic compensated respiratory acidosis.
2. Case 53, page 165. Metabolic alkalosis.
3. Case 54, page 167. Acute respiratory alkalosis.
4. Case 90, page 307. Type 1 respiratory failure.
5. Case 93, page 319. Type 2 respiratory failure.

Case 37

Polyuria and Lithium Toxicity

A 48-year-old woman who was known to be depressed for the past 5 years presented with polyuria. Drug history was not available. Physical examination was unremarkable.

Fasting blood glucose	5.2 mmol/l
Na	132 mmol/l
K	3.6 mmol/l
Urea	6.0 mmol/l
Creatinine	112 µmol/l
Corrected calcium	3.1 mmol/l
PO_4	0.5 mmol/l
TSH	2.1 U/l

The patient declined a water deprivation test

What two investigations are required to identify the cause of her polyuria?

A. Renal ultrasound
B. Intravenous urography
C. Anti-diuretic hormone (ADH)
D. Glucose tolerance test
E. Parathyroid hormone (PTH)
F. Renal biopsy
G. Serum compliment
H. Lithium levels
I. Creatinine clearance

Answers: (E, H)

DISCUSSION

This depressed patient is on lithium therapy. Her serum lithium level was 0.7 mmol/l. Hypercalcaemia can cause nephrogenic diabetes insipidus and produce symptoms of polyuria. The hypercalcaemia may be due to hyperparathyroidism or chronic lithium therapy.

Lithium Toxicity

Lithium carbonate or citrate is the main therapeutic agent for the prophylactic treatment of bipolar affective disorders. It is given orally and rapidly absorbed from the gastrointestinal tract. The elimination is mainly through the kidneys where > 95 per cent is excreted. Its clinical effects appear after about 10 days. The therapeutic levels are 0.5 - 1.0 mmol/l; levels > 2.0 mmol/l are toxic.

Clinical features of acute lithium toxicity

- Dizziness
- Blurred vision
- Coarse tremor
- Ataxia and dysarthria
- Eventually delirium and convulsions

Chronic side effects of lithium

These can occur even with normal blood levels:

- Weight gain and increased appetite
- Gastrointestinal symptoms
- Fine tremor
- Hypothyroidism, hyperthyroidism
- Lithium induced nephrogenic diabetes insipidus
- Hypercalcaemia: hypercalcaemia may occur especially if the patient is also on thiazide diuretics. In lithium therapy hypercalcaemia is associated with hypocalciuria and a normal or elevated PTH. A 24 hr urinary calcium may help. It is, therefore, difficult to diagnose primary hyperparathyroidism in any lithium-treated patient, although very high calcium levels (> 3.0 mmol/l) are more likely to be due to hyperparathyroidism.

Case 38

Metabolic Acidosis with High Anion Gap, Lactic Acidosis, Salicylate Poisoning

A 72-year-old woman was brought to the A and E department having been found by her husband to be drowsy and hyperventilating. She was a type 2 diabetic for the last 2 years and had a myocardial infarct 5 years ago, which was complicated by acute pulmonary oedema. She was on aspirin 75 mg od, ramipril 10 mg od, furosemide 40 mg od, simvastatin 40 mg od, atenolol 50 mg od and metformin 500 mg tds. On examination, she was rousable to painful stimuli and had no signs of neck rigidity. She was hyperventilating with a respiratory rate of 28 per minute. The heart rate was regular at 88 bpm and blood pressure 110/70 mm Hg. The pupils were equal and reactive to light. Doll's eye movement was present and there was no papilloedema.

Na	144 mmol/l
K	5.4 mmol/l
Urea	12 mmol/l
Creatinine	144 µmol/l
Glucose	14 mmol/l
Chloride	98 mmol/l
HCO_3	10 mmol/l
Hb	12.0 g/dl
WBC	7.0 x 10^9/l
Platelets	240 x 10^9/l
Urinalysis	protein positive glucose positive ketone negative

What are the two most important diagnostic tests?

A. CT head
B. MRI brain scan with contrast

C. Serum lactate and salicylate levels
D. EEG
E. Lumbar puncture
F. Serum metformin levels
G. Fibrin degradation products
H. Ammonium chloride loading test
I. Arterial blood gases
J. Coagulation screen

Answer (C, I)

DISCUSSION

This patient has a severe metabolic acidosis with a high anion gap (see below). An increased anion gap is due to the accumulation of organic acids or lactate, as in the following conditions:

- Diabetic ketoacidosis due to insulin deficiency
- Salicylate poisoning
- Lactic acidosis (see below)
- Renal failure (accumulation of sulphate and phosphate)

The anion gap for this patient is calculated as follows:

Anion gap $= \{Na + K\} - \{HCO_3 + Cl\}$
$= \{144 + 5.4\} - \{10 + 98\}$
$= 41$

Normal anion gap $= 12\text{-}16$

In this patient, there is no ketonuria to suggest diabetic ketoacidosis. Salicylate levels need to be checked to exclude aspirin overdose. She has type 2 diabetes and metformin can cause lactic acidosis in the presence of heart failure and renal impairment.

Lactic acidosis

Lactic acidosis may be divided into type A and type B.

Type A lactic acidosis is due to anaerobic metabolism in tissues such as in:

- Cardiac arrest (acidosis worsens cardiac function and causes vasoconstriction)
- Hypotension
- Sepsis
- Overdose (phenobarbitone, alcohol)

Type B lactic acidosis is seen in:

- Metformin (especially in presence of heart failure, renal disease or hepatic dysfunction)
- Hepatic dysfunction (decreased metabolism of lactate)
- Insulin deficiency which causes lactic acidosis due to decreased pyruvate dehydrogenase activity

LINKS TO BOOK ONE

1. Case 47, page 144. Chronic compensated respiratory acidosis.
2. Case 53, page 165. Metabolic alkalosis.
3. Case 54, page 167. Acute respiratory alkalosis.
4. Case 90, page 307. Type 1 respiratory failure.
5. Case 93, page 319. Type 2 respiratory failure.

Case 39

Tumour Lysis Syndrome

A 27-year-old leukaemic patient received his first course of chemotherapy and became very ill two days later.

Na	142 mmol/l
K	7.3 mmol/l
Urea	36.5 mmol/l
Creatinine	199 µmol/l
PO_4	1.8 mmol/l

What is the cause of his renal failure?

A. Tumour lysis syndrome
B. Acute glomerulonephritis
C. Acute interstitial nephritis
D. Pre-renal uraemia
E. Obstructive nephropathy

Answer (A)

DISCUSSION

Tumour Lysis Syndrome

Tumour lysis syndrome from chemotherapy is fortunately rare nowadays due to the increased awareness of this condition and appropriate prophylactic measures being taken prior to cancer chemotherapy. Tumour lysis syndrome may arise following chemotherapy of tumours that have a very fast cellular turn over such as B-cell or T-cell acute lymphatic leukaemias. Tumour lysis results in a high phosphate and potassium levels, which are released from damaged cells. The high phosphate mops up the calcium leading to hypocalcaemia. Treatment is difficult once the condition has developed and the urgent correction of metabolic disturbances may require dialysis.

The following measures are essential to prevent tumour lysis syndrome:

- Do not start chemotherapy unless the serum uric acid is normal
- Treat hyperuricaemia with allopurinol
- Ensure adequate hydration
- Monitor serum U and E, calcium, phosphate and uric acid
- Alkalinization of urine
- Injections of encapsulated uricase, which degrades insoluble uric acid to the soluble allantoin, have also been advocated in the acute treatment of severe hyperuricaemia.

Case 40

Sideroblastic Anaemia and Iron Deficiency

An 85-year-old man was referred for investigation of anaemia. He has diverticular disease and an active duodenal ulcer in the past. He consumed about 2 pints of beer a day.

Hb	7.0 g/dl
WBC	$4.6 \times 10^9/l$
Platelets	$180 \times 10^9/l$
MCV	114 fl
Iron	4 μmol/l (ref 13 - 32)
TIBC	76 μmol/l (ref 42 - 80)
Serum folate	28 nmol/l (ref 5 - 40)
Vitamin B_{12}	290 pmol/l (ref 130 - 660)
TSH	3.5 mU/l
Blood film	hypochromia and macrocytosis

Bone marrow aspirate showed absent stainable iron stores and ring sideroblasts.

What is the diagnosis?

A. Sideroblastic anaemia on the background of iron deficiency
B. Iron deficiency anaemia being treated with iron therapy
C. Anaemia due to occult malignancy
D. Anaemia related to alcohol
E. Myelodysplastic anaemia

Answer: (A)

DISCUSSION

Sideroblastic Anaemia

This is a difficult case. The differential features of iron deficiency and sideroblastic anaemia are shown below:

	Iron deficiency anaemia	**Sideroblastic anaemia**
Serum iron	↓	↑
Total iron binding capacity	↑	Normal
Serum ferritin	↓	↑
Iron in erythroblasts	Absent	Ring forms
Iron in marrow	Absent	Present

This patient has features of iron deficiency (i.e. low serum iron and a absent stainable iron in the bone marrow). There were also ring sideroblasts in the bone marrow. Ring sideroblasts are the result of disordered haem synthesis, which leads to the accumulation of iron granules in the mitochondria of erythroblasts. These granules are arranged in a ring around the nucleus and can be demonstrated with Pearl's reaction.

Causes of sideroblastic anaemia

I. Inherited
   a. Sex linked

II. Acquired
   a. Primary – a type of myelodysplastic syndrome
   b. Secondary due to
      - Alcohol
      - Drugs (e.g. isoniazid)
      - Lead poisoning
      - Myeloid leukaemia and other myeloproliferative disorders
      - Chronic inflammatory disease (e.g. rheumatoid disease)

Myelodysplastic syndrome

This is a group of bone marrow disorders due to an acquired defect in bone marrow stem cells resulting in quantitative and qualitative abnormalities of erythrocytes, leucocytes and platelets, as well as a tendency for leukaemic transformation.

Clinical features of myelodysplastic syndrome

The patient is commonly elderly with one or more of the following features:

- Anaemia
- Bleeding (reduced platelets)

- Infection (neutropenia)
- Transformation to chronic myelomonocytic leukaemia
- Acute myeloblastic leukaemia may occur in up to 30 per cent of patients

Classification of myelodysplastic syndrome

- Refractory anaemia, RA.
- Refractory anaemia with ringed sideroblasts (> 15% ringed sideroblasts), RARS.
- Refractory anaemia with excess blast cells (bone marrow blast cell count between 5-20%), RAEB.
- Refractory anaemia with excess blast cells in transformation (blast count 20-30%), RAEB-t.
- Chronic myelomonocytic leukaemia, CMML.

Bone marrow

- Increased cellularity despite pancytopenia
- Ring sideroblasts present in all types
- Increased blasts in RAEB and RAEB-t
- Abnormal morphology of granulocyte and megakaryocyte precursors

Treatment

I. Bone marrow blast count < 5 per cent
- Conservative ('wait and see' policy)
- Supportive measures for infection, bleeding and anaemia
- May consider G-CSF (granulocyte colony stimulating factor)

II. Bone marrow blast count > 5 per cent
- Conservative for frail elderly
- Refer to specialist centre for intensive chemotherapy or bone marrow transplant

LINKS TO BOOK ONE

1. Case 6, page 16. Myelodysplasia.

Case 41

von Willebrand's Disease

A 5-year-old boy underwent circumcision, but post-operatively the bleeding did not stop.

Hb	10.2 g/dl
WBC	7.1 x 10^9/l
Platelets	179 x 10^9/l
Blood film	no abnormality
Bleeding time	10.6 minutes
PT	14 seconds (patient)
	12 seconds (control)
APTT	52 seconds (patient)
	36 seconds (control)

What is the most appropriate therapeutic intervention?

A. Intravenous vitamin K
B. Fresh frozen plasma
C. Cryoprecipitate
D. von Willebrand's factor concentrate
E. Intravenous calcium chloride

Answer (D)

DISCUSSION

von Willebrand's Disease

Factor VIII consists of:

- A molecule with coagulant activity called VIII:C which is synthesized by the liver. Its production is controlled by genes located on the X chromosome.
- von Willebrand factor (vWF) is synthesized by endothelial cells. Its synthesis is controlled by genes on chromosome 12.

The functions of vWF are:

- Stabilization of factor VIII:C in the circulation and preventing its degradation
- Promotion of platelet-endothelial interaction

von Willebrand's disease (vWD) is characterized by deficiency or abnormality of von Willebrand factor. Consequently, there is impaired platelet function and factor VIII:C deficiency.

Platelet aggregation studies

The platelets fail to aggregate in contact with ristocetin in patients with von Willebrand's disease and Bernard-Soulier syndrome. Bernard-Soulier syndrome is inherited as an autosomal dominant disorder and presents with giant platelets and there may be a low platelet count.

Inheritance of vWD

von Willebrand's disease may be inherited as:

1. Autosomal dominant, which usually presents with a bleeding tendency and is similar to mild haemophilia, including:
   - Bleeding after trauma or surgery
   - Epistaxis
   - Menorrhagia
   - Rarely haemarthrosis
2. Autosomal recessive (i.e. both parents are haematologically normal), which has the severest presentation, including:
   - Haemarthrosis
   - Muscle haematoma

Table 41.1: Differences between haemophilia and von Willebrand's disease

	Haemophilia	**von Willebrand's disease**
Bleeding time	Normal	Prolonged
Prothrombin time	Normal	Normal
APPT	Normal	Normal or prolonged
VIII:C	Reduced	Reduced
vWF	Normal	Reduced

The manifestations of Vitamin K deficiency

Adult vitamin K deficiency occurs in malabsorption syndromes, liver disease and obstructive jaundice. There is competitive antagonism between warfarin and vitamin K: prothrombin time and APTT are both prolonged.

Common Features of Warfarin Overdose

- Bruising
- Haematuria
- Gastrointestinal haemorrhage
- Cerebral haemorrhage

British Society of Haematology recommendations for warfarin over anticoagulation (1990).

- Life threatening haemorrhage: give vitamin K 5 mg IV + fresh frozen plasma (or if available concentrate of clotting factors II, IX, X, VII).
- Less severe haemorrhage (haematuria or epistaxis): withhold warfarin for one or more days; and consider vitamin K 0.5 – 2mg IV.
- INR > 4.5 without haemorrhage: withhold warfarin for 1 or 2 days and then review.

Case 42

Deep Vein Thrombosis

A 50-year-old man presented to an acute medical ward with a left hemiparesis. CT brain scan showed an ischaemic lesion in the right parietal lobe. Aspirin 150 mg od was started. He was assessed by the stroke team and found to have no problems with speech, swallowing or vision. Two weeks later, he developed swelling of the left leg, which extended up to the groin.

What is the most appropriate management?

A. Intravenous benzylpenicillin and flucloxacillin
B. Anticoagulation with heparin followed by warfarin
C. TED stockings
D. Leg elevation
E. Intravenous fluids and increased aspirin to 300 mg od

Answer (B)

DISCUSSION

Risk factors for deep vein thrombosis

- Immobility
- Postoperative (especially pelvic or orthopaedic surgery)
- Cardiac failure
- Recent myocardial infarction
- Previous deep vein thrombosis
- Stroke
- Infections
- Dehydration
- Malignancy
- Pregnancy and postpartum

- Drugs such steroids, oral contraceptive pills
- Inflammatory bowel disease
- Homocystinuria
- Thrombophilia

Thrombophilia

- Anti-thrombin III deficiency
- Protein C deficiency
- Protein S deficiency
- Factor V Leiden

Factor V Leiden

- Factor V is a cofactor for thrombin generation (a coagulation factor).
- Factor V is inactivated by protein C
- Factor V Leiden is found in 3-5 per cent of the population, but in up to 20 per cent of patients with venous thrombosis.
- Factor V Leiden has a single amino acid substitution (arginine is replaced by glutamine in position 506), which alters its binding site for protein C. In this way factor V Leiden is less susceptible to inactivation by protein C.
- Factor V Leiden enhances thrombosis in the presence of other risk factors (see those listed under risk factors for DVT).

LINKS TO BOOK ONE

1. Case 26, page 75. Heparin induced thrombocytopenia.
2. Case 28, page 85. Thrombophilia.
3. Case 42, page 130. Polycythaemia vera.
4. Case 60, page 191. Thrombocytosis and essential thrombocythaemia.

Case 43

Infectious Mononucleosis

A 20-year-old college student recently returned from Malta where he had spent two months on a working holiday. He complained of sore throat, fever, joint pains and generalised aching in the past one week. On examination, his temperature was 38.5° Celsius, the throat was inflamed, and there were tender small lymph nodes in the neck, axillae and groins. The spleen was just palpable.

Hb	10.3 g/dl
WBC	14 x 10^9/l
Platelets	186 x 10^9/l
Neutrophils	40 per cent
Lymphocytes	50 per cent
Monocytes	8 per cent
Blood film	atypical lymphocytes, no blast cells

What is the most likely diagnosis?

A. Brucellosis
B. Toxoplasmosis
C. Infectious mononucleosis
D. Q fever
E. Cytomegalovirus infection

Answer (C)

DISCUSSION

Infectious Mononucleosis

Infectious mononucleosis is caused by the Epstein-Barr virus (EBV), which is an enveloped DNA herpesvirus. Transmission is through intimate contact with the saliva of an infected person and hence the term 'kissing disease'. It is a common illness during adolescence or young adulthood.

Pathophysiology

The incubation time of EBV infection is between 4 and 6 weeks. The virus infects the oral epithelial cells and B-lymphocytes. These lymphocytes then enter the reticuloendothelial system to mount an immunological response, giving rise to the clinical manifestations of the disease. Although the symptoms resolve in 1 or 2 months, the virus remains dormant in the body (carrier state). A few of these carriers may go on to develop Burkitt's lymphoma and nasopharyngeal carcinoma. When symptoms last for more than 6 months, the illness is called chronic EBV infection. In chronic disease, patients present with tiredness, low-grade fever, headache, and sore throat.

Clinical manifestations of infectious mononucleosis

I. Prodromal symptoms
   - Malaise
   - Anorexia
   - Fatigue
   - Headache
   - Fever

II. Symptoms
   - Fever
   - Sore throat
   - Swollen lymph glands

III. Signs
   - Lymphadenopathy (anterior and posterior cervical chains)
   - Palatal petechiae may be present.
   - Splenomegaly (resolves by 4 weeks)
   - Temperature may be as high as 40° Celsius

IV. Less common features
   - Upper airway compromise
   - Rash
   - Hepatomegaly
   - Jaundice
   - Eyelid oedema

Diagnosis

- Clinical diagnosis: characteristic triad of fever, pharyngitis and lymphadenopathy.
- Increased blood lymphocytes (atypical lymphocyte count > 10%).
- Positive Paul-Bunnell heterophile antibody test. These antibodies develop one week after the onset of symptoms. If the heterophil antibody test is negative and infectious mononucleosis is still suspected, serum for viral capsid antigen and EBV nuclear antigen should be sent.

Management of infectious mononucleosis

- The treatment is mainly supportive.
- Aspirin should be avoided as it can precipitate Reye's syndrome.
- Patients should be advised to avoid vigorous activity for 3 to 4 weeks to avoid the risk of splenic rupture.
- Ampicillin and amoxycillin should be avoided as patients may develop a rash with these drugs.

Differential diagnosis of infectious mononucleosis

- Chronic fatigue syndrome
- Cytomegalovirus (sore throat is less severe and lymphadenopathy may be minimal or absent)
- Adenovirus infection
- *Toxoplasma gondii* (sore throat is less severe)

Atypical lymphocytes

Atypical lymphocytes are activated T-cells with increased cytoplasm and less mature nuclear material. These atypical lymphocytes may be seen in other conditions, albeit in fewer numbers. In addition to EBV infections, the conditions in which atypical lymphocytes might be seen include:

- Cytomegalovirus (However, pharyngitis is usually not a feature of CMV infection or in toxoplasmosis)
- Toxoplasmosis
- Acute HIV infection
- Hepatitis

- Rubella
- Roseola
- Lymphoproliferative disorders

Complications of EBV infection

- Reactivation of the viral infection
- Lymphoma: EBV causes inappropriate lymphocyte proliferation, but only a small proportion of EBV-associated lymphocyte proliferation results in lymphoma which may be:
  - Non-Hodgkin's Lymphoma
  - Burkitt's lymphoma
  - Post-transplant lymphoproliferative disease associated with immuno-suppressive therapy.
- Nasopharyngeal carcinoma
- Hairy leukoplakia. This presents as corrugated white lesions mostly on the lateral border of the tongue. Biopsy is needed to confirm the diagnosis. The appearance of hairy leukoplakia should alert the clinician to exclude HIV infection.

False positive heterophile antibody tests

- Rubella
- Malaria
- Serum hepatitis
- Systemic lupus erythematosus
- Leukaemia
- Pancreatic cancer

LINKS TO BOOK ONE

1. Case 92, page 315. Chronic lymphatic leukaemia.
2. Case 95, page 330. Chronic myeloid leukaemia.

Case 44

Methyldopa Haemolysis Anaemia

A 74-year-old woman attended the A and E department because of excessive tiredness and exertional shortness of breath. She had been a hypertensive patient for the last ten years and was treated with one medication, but did not remember its name. She was a non-smoker and did not consume alcohol.

Na	135 mmol/l
K	5.2 mmol/l
Urea	6.5 mmol/l
Creatinine	112 μmol/l
Bilirubin	52 μmol/l
ALT	18 U/l
ALP	144 U/l
Total protein	7.4 g/l
Albumin	3.2 g/l
CK	170 U/l
Troponin T	< 0.01 μg/l
Hb	7.2 g/dl
WBC	11.2×10^9/l
Platelets	262×10^9/l
MCV	110 fl
MCHC	31%
Reticulocyte count	16%
Direct Coombs' test	Positive
CXR	Cardiomegaly but no pulmonary congestion
ECG	Sinus rhythm with left ventricular strain

The provisional diagnosis was a haemolytic anaemia, probably drug induced.

Which one of the following drugs she may be using?

A. Bendroflumethiazide
B. Nifedipine
C. Captopril
D. Reserpine
E. Methyldopa

Answer (E)

DISCUSSION

Haemolytic Anaemia

This patient has hyperbilirubinaemia without evidence of hepatocellular damage or obstructive jaundice. The most likely diagnostic possibility is haemolytic anaemia. This is supported by:

- Reticulocytosis
- Positive direct Coombs' test

Reticulocytosis indicates rapid turn over of the erythrocytic cells in the bone marrow which occur in:

- Haemolysis
- Active bleeding
- Treatment phase of anaemia secondary to deficiency of iron, vitamin B_{12} and folate

Markers of haemolysis

- Unconjugated hyperbilirubinaemia
- Excessive urobilinogen in the urine
- Intravascular haemolysis is supported by:
  - Raised plasma levels of free haemoglobin
  - Reduced or absent haptoglobin and haemopexin
  - Positive methaemoglobinaemia (Schumm's test)
  - Haemosiderinuria
  - Haemoglobinuria
- Reticulocytosis
- The blood film may also show abnormal red cells such as: spherocytosis, schistocytes, target cells and elliptocytosis. Spherocytosis are small rounded red cells that occur in congenital spherocytic anaemias, autoimmune haemolytic anaemia (AIHA). Schistocytes are broken red cells and usually seen in disseminated intravascular haemolysis (DIC) and

mechanical destruction of red cells such as in haemolysis due to prosthetic cardiac valves. Target cells are frequently seen in alcoholic liver disease and thalassaemia. Elliptocytes are features of congenital elliptocytosis.

- Bone marrow hyperplasia
- Red cell survival studies with ^{51}Cr labelled red cells may be required

Autoimmune haemolytic anaemia (AIHA)

Antibody mediated haemolytic destruction of red cells is characterized by a positive direct Coomb's test. AIHA is classified into "warm" and "cold", depending on the temperature at which the antibodies attach themselves to the red cells.

Warm AIHA

Warm AIHA refers to red cell destruction by antibodies operating at body temperature. These antibodies are usually IgG and the causes are:

- Idiopathic
- Lymphoproliferative disease (lymphoma or chronic lymphatic leukaemia)
- Some solid cancers
- Collagen diseases such as systemic lupus erythematosus
- Drugs such as methyldopa

Cold AIHA

Cold AIHA refers to red cell destruction by antibodies operating at temperatures less than 37° Celsius. They are usually of the IgM type. The usual causes are:

- Infectious diseases such as
  - Mycoplasma
  - Epstein-Barr virus
  - Cytomegalovirus
- Lymphomas particularly histiocytic types
- Paroxysmal Cold Haemoglobinuria
- Idiopathic

The patient may suffer from acrocyanosis and Raynaud's phenomenon due to agglutination of red cells when the peripheral parts (hands and feet) are exposed to cold temperatures. When these red cells return to higher core temperatures, they may undergo intravascular haemolysis.

Drug induced haemolysis

Drugs can cause haemolysis via different mechanisms including:

a. Autoimmune haemolysis such as: methyldopa, levodopa, and mefenamic acid.

   This type of anaemia usually requires prolonged exposure to the drug (3-6 months) and the Coombs' test is positive. The anaemia is extravascular.

b. Immune complex formation: isoniazid, rifampicin, amidopyrine and sulfonamides. The anaemia is intravascular and could occur after low dosages, but needs second or subsequent exposures.

c. Hapten-membrane association: Penicillin and cefalosporins. The anaemia is extravascular and occurs after large doses have been used for extended periods of time as in the treatment of bacterial endocarditis.

Case 45

Carcinoid Syndrome

A 52-year-old man was admitted for investigation of diarrhoea and abdominal pain. He had loose stools for the last 3 months and opened his bowel 3-4 times daily, but there was no rectal bleeding or blood stained stools. The abdominal pain was colicky, occurring every few days, lasting for a few hours, and not related to bowel actions. His appetite was poor. There was no recent antibiotic use or foreign travel. Two weeks ago, he suddenly developed a dry cough and breathlessness. There was no fever or haemoptysis. The General Practitioner had prescribed beclomethasone inhaler 200 μg bd and salbutamol inhaler 200 μg qds.

On examination, he was emaciated and had bluish-reddish pigmentation on the cheeks. On closer inspection, these were telangiectasiae. On direct questioning, he admitted to regular attacks of facial flushing. There was no lymphadenopathy, but liver was enlarged 4 cm below the costal margin. Chest examination revealed bilateral expiratory wheezes. The heart rate was regular at 88 bpm and blood pressure 120/70 mm Hg. There was a soft systolic murmur at the left upper sternal edge.

Stool cultures (three samples)	negative
Stools for *Clostridium difficile* toxin	negative
Coeliac disease antibody screen	negative
Gastroscopy	normal
Duodenal biopsy	normal mucosa
Barium enema	few diverticula at sigmoid colon
Colonoscopy	normal

Hb	10.4 g/dl
WBC	$5.4 \times 10^9/l$
Neutrophils	60%

Lymphocyte	35%
Monocyte	5%
Platelets	$235 \times 10^9/l$
ALT	41 U/l
ALP	311 U/l
Albumin	30 g/l
Total protein	69 g/l
INR	2.1

What investigation is likely to be diagnostic?

A. Barium meal
B. D – Xylose test
C. CT scan of the abdomen
D. Echocardiography
E. Urinary 5-hydroxy-indole acetic acid assay

Answer (E)

DISCUSSION

The combination of facial flushing, skin pigmentation, diarrhoea, wheezy chest and cardiac murmur suggested the diagnosis of carcinoid syndrome, which was confirmed by subsequent investigations.

Carcinoid syndrome

The annual incidence of carcinoid syndrome is about 1 in 500,000 of the population. Carcinoid syndrome occurs in about 10 per cent of patients with carcinoid tumours. These tumours are capable of producing one or more of the following chemical substances, which give rise to the clinical features of carcinoid syndrome:

- Serotonin (5-hydroxytryptamine; 5-HT) synthesized from the amino acid tryptophan precipitates the symptoms of diarrhoea and bronchoconstriction. It is metabolized to 5-hydroxy-indole acetic acid (5-HIAA), which is excreted in urine.
- Substance P induces flushing.
- Histamine probably causes a wheal-like flush (seen with gastric carcinoid tumours).

The most common sites for carcinoid tumours are the appendix and rectum. Other sites include:

- Small intestine (ileum, appendix)

- Embryonic foregut derivatives (bronchus, stomach, thyroid, pancreas)
- Teratomas (ovarian or testicular)

The majority of primary tumours originate from the small bowel. 5-HT is metabolized in the liver and hence, mid-gut tumours cause symptoms only after metastastic spread usually to the liver. Primary carcinoid tumours from the bronchial tree constitute about 10 per cent of all carcinoid tumours, but they tend to be chemically inactive and present with haemoptysis, focal wheezing and recurrent chest infections.

Clinical manifestations

- Flushing of the head and upper thorax is the characteristic feature. Initially they come in paroxysms and are associated with tachycardia, hypotension, and increased skin temperature. The duration is only a few minutes to begin with, but as the disease progresses symptoms may become continuous. Precipitating factors include alcohol, stress or emotion.
- Chronically reddened and cyanotic facial hue
- Telangiectasiae
- Migratory wheal-like areas of flushing
- Profuse secretary diarrhoea
- Wheezing
- Weight loss (poor dietary intake and malabsorption)
- Pellagra (nicotinamide deficiency is due to excessive conversion of 5-hydroxytryptophan into 5-HT)
- Cardiac valve abnormalities (endocardial fibrosis). These lesions almost always occur on the right side of the heart. The most common lesions are tricuspid incompetence and pulmonary stenosis. Left-sided valve damage occurs in bronchial carcinoid.
- Other endocrine syndromes: Cushing's syndrome (ectopic ACTH-secretion), acromegaly (ectopic GHRH), Type 1 Multiple Endocrine Neoplasia (Wermer's syndrome).

Investigations

- Diagnostic - Elevation in urinary 5-HIAA
- Computed tomographic (CT) scanning or abdominal ultrasonography

- Chest radiographs and CT scans of the chest
- ^{123}I-iodobenzylguanidine (MIBG) scan
- ^{111}Indium labelled octreotide scan (80-90% of carcinoid tumours display somatostatin receptors)

Management

- Somatostatin analogues are the first-line treatment: octreotide (subcutaneous injections tds) or lanreotide (subcutaneous injection every 14 days) are indicated for flushing. The adverse effects are hypoglycaemia, gallstones, and steatorrhoea. Octreotide is also life saving in carcinoid crisis.
- Codeine and loperamide to control diarrhoea. *If no response somatostatin analogues can be used to control diarrhoea.*
- Alpha interferon
- Hepatic artery embolization of metastastic deposits in the liver
- Nicotinamide for pellagra
- Antihistamines may be useful in histamine-related tumours
- Surgery (tumour debulking)

False-positive results with urinary 5-HIAA

- Foods such as bananas, pineapples, avocados, plums, chocolates
- Paracetamol
- Fluorouracil
- Chlorpromazine
- Levodopa
- Methysergide
- Caffeine

Differential diagnosis of flushing

- Idiopathic anaphylaxis
- Alcohol ingestion
- Post-menopause
- Hyperthyroidism
- Vipoma
- Medullary thyroid carcinoma
- Systemic mastocytosis

Case 46

Malabsorption: Intestinal TB and Coeliac Disease

A 26-year-old refugee from the Middle East presented to the medical out-patient department complaining of backache, frequent loose stools that were pale and difficult to flush and 5 kg weight loss. He has chronic backache for which he was taking ibuprofen 200 mg tds. He had arrived in the United Kingdom two months ago. At the age of 20 years, he received twelve months of chemotherapy for pulmonary tuberculosis. He was currently unemployed, smoked 20 cigarettes daily, but was teetotal. On examination, there was impaired percussion note at the apex of the left lung with tracheal shift to the left. There was no finger clubbing, ankle oedema or hepatosplenomegaly.

Hb	8.2 g/dl
WBC	10.2×10^9/l
Platelets	340×10^9/l
ESR	18 mm/h
MCV	111 fl
MCHC	31.3 g/dl
Vitamin B_{12}	230 pmol/l
Serum folate	1.2 nmol/l
Na	132 mmol/l
K	3.3 mmol/l
Urea	2.4 mmol/l
Creatinine	96 µmol/l
Glucose	5.2 mmol/l
Albumin	30 g/l
Globulin	24 g/l
Corrected calcium	1.8 mmol/l
PO_4	0.9 mmol/l

ALP	315 U/l
Chest X-ray	Old fibrotic lesion in the apex of the left lung

Which one of following statements is correct?

A. These symptoms are suggestive of inflammatory bowel disease
B. Giardiasis is unlikely
C. D-xylose absorption test will uncover the cause of his diarrhoea
D. Coeliac disease needs to be excluded
E. Barium meal and follow through should be the first screening test

Answer (D)

DISCUSSION

- The macrocytic anaemia, low serum folate, hypoalbuminaemia, and hypocalcaemia suggests malabsorption syndrome. The normal ESR and absence of bloody diarrhoea make the diagnosis of inflammatory bowel disease unlikely.
- Giardiasis is a distinctive possibility as this protozoan is quite common in Middle Eastern countries, but intestinal lymphomas are uncommon.
- *The D-xylose absorption test is abnormal in malabsorption due to small bowel pathology, but does not provide a specific diagnosis.*
- The chronic ingestion of ibuprofen and other NSAIDs can produce NSAID enteropathy, but this is usually asymptomatic, although inflammatory changes and increase in mucosal permeability can lead to hypoalbuminaemia and iron deficiency. Small and large bowel ulcerations in NSAID enteropathy can also lead to fibrosis and the subsequent formation of diaphragmatic strictures (so called "diaphragm disease"), which can present with obstructive symptoms and then require operative intervention.
- Taking into account this patient's past medical history of pulmonary TB, one has to think of intestinal tuberculosis as a cause of his symptoms. However, the normal ESR and the absence of constitutional symptoms make this diagnosis less likely.

- Coeliac disease is less common in someone from the Middle East but can be excluded relatively easily by:
  - Measuring anti-tissue transglutaminase, gliadin, or endomysial antibodies
  - Endoscopic duodenal biopsy
- In this patient the diagnosis of coeliac disease was confirmed by serology and histology.

The essential investigations are

- Gastroscopy and duodenal biopsy
- Coeliac disease antibodies
- Stool examination for *Giardia lamblia*
- Stool culture for *Mycobacterium bacilli*
- Barium meal and follow through
- X-ray of the spine
- Assessment of the malnutrition resulting from malabsorption (serum ferritin, folate, B_{12}, and vitamin D assay)
- If the diagnosis of tuberculous enteritis is still a possibility, one should arrange stool cultures for TB, CT scan of the abdomen (may show mesenteric lymphadenopathy, thickening of the colonic wall and ascites). Colonoscopy and biopsy may confirm colonic TB and it may be possible to negotiate the ileocaecal valve and gain access to the terminal ileum.

Coeliac disease

Coeliac disease is a chronic inflammatory disease of the small intestine, which improves morphologically when gluten is removed from the diet. It is also called gluten-sensitive enteropathy or non-tropical sprue. It can affect people of all ages. In the United Kingdom, the prevalence is estimated to be 1 in 300 people. The peak incidence in adulthood is in the third decade. The main features are of malabsorption and malnutrition including:

- General lassitude.
- Diarrhoea, but this is not present in all the patients (they may present with anaemia only).
- Iron and folate deficiency.
- Vitamin D and K deficiency.
- Other features include reduced fertility, psychological disturbances, or neurological deficits such as ataxia.

- Dermatitis herpetiformis may be seen in 2 to 5 per cent of patients with coeliac disease. It is an itchy blistering skin eruption, which frequently affects the knees, elbows, buttocks and back. The presence of IgA at the dermo-epidermal junction of uninvolved skin on biopsy confirms the diagnosis.
- The malnutrition and malabsorption features of coeliac disease in childhood will affect growth leading to failure to thrive and short stature. Other siblings of the patient should also be screened.

Diagnostic investigation

- Serological screening tests can be performed for antibodies to gliadin and endomysium. More recently, IgA anti-Tissue Transglutaminase (tTG) antibodies can be measured easily and cheaply, being present in 90 per cent of patients with untreated disease, and are relatively specific.
- Intestinal biopsy from the distal duodenum or jejunum. There are characteristic histological changes including loss of height of the villi, crypt hyperplasia, chronic inflammatory cell infiltration of the lamina propria, lymphocytic infiltration of the epithelium, and a decrease in the epithelial surface-cell height. Improvement or reversal of these histological changes with a follow-up biopsy obtained 4 to 6 months after starting treatment with a gluten-free diet confirms the diagnosis. A formal gluten challenge test followed by small intestinal biopsy can be done. A small intestinal biopsy is mandatory to confirm the diagnosis. However, it is now acceptable to take only an initial biopsy in patients who have typical histological features, as long as they have positive antibodies to gliadin and endomysium and experience symptomatic improvement on the withdrawal of dietary gluten.

Supportive investigations

- Full blood count, vitamin B_{12}, folate and iron
- Red cell morphology and blood film: a dimorphic blood picture may be seen in patients who develop both iron and folate deficiencies.
- Total serum protein and serum albumin (protein losing enteropathy)

- Liver function tests and bone profile (calcium, phosphate) to screen for osteomalacia
- Small intestinal barium studies show malabsorption pattern: dilatation of the jejunal loops, loss of the normal feathery appearance in the jejunum, flocculation of the barium suspension, thickening of the mucosal fold pattern and delayed transit (Figure 46.1). These changes are not diagnostic of coeliac disease as they may be present in other conditions.
- Barium follow through can be performed in sequence to barium meal and metoclopramide can be used to speed up the procedure. Barium follow through is also useful to exclude other causes of malabsorption and diarrhoea, and for diagnosing complications of coeliac disease, such as strictures and small bowel lymphoma. Small bowel enema is preferred by many centres over the barium follow through, and it is obtained by passing a fine tube into the duodenum and barium sulphate is followed by a propellant such as methylcellulose suspension.

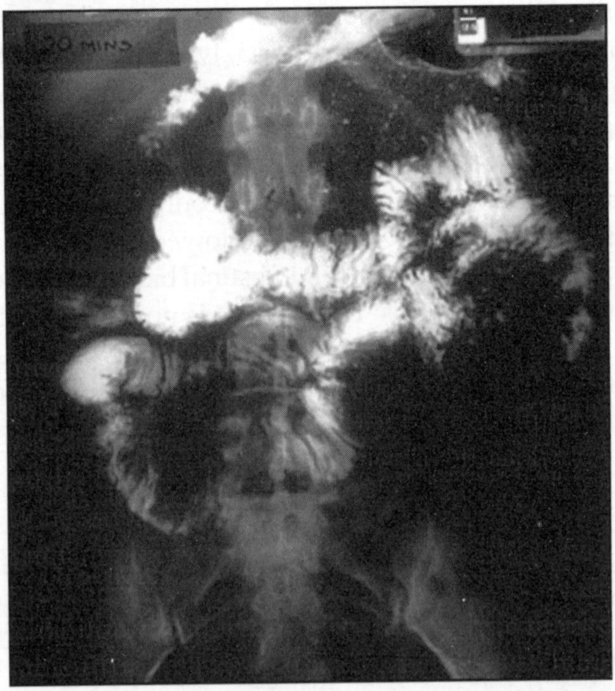

Figure 46.1: Barium follow through of a 78-year-old patient with malabsorption due to coeliac disease

Treatment of coeliac disease

- Gluten free diet. Histological improvement usually takes many months to occur. The dietary restrictions are needed life long.
- Treatment of dietary deficiencies of iron, folic acid, calcium and vitamin B_{12}.
- Pneumococcal vaccine is recommended because of the hyposplenism in coeliac disease makes these patients liable to infections by encapsulated bacteria (pneumococcus, haemophilus influenzae, and *Neisseria meningitidis*).
- Information and support. It is crucial that all these patients are given proper dietary advice and see a dietician. They should be provided with leaflets explaining all aspects of the disease and encouraged to join the coeliac disease society.
- Follow-up is needed at six to twelve monthly intervals. This should include clinical and nutritional state assessments. Anti-tissue Transglutaminase (tTG) antibody titres are monitored to assess treatment response. A repeat small intestinal biopsy after initiating treatment is not performed routinely unless the condition is resistant to treatment or complications suspected. Life long follow-up is recommended because of long-term complications, such as lymphoma and bone disease.
- Dapsone is the drug of choice for dermatitis herpetiformis. The side effects of dapsone include a dose-dependent haemolytic anaemia, methaemoglobinaemia and headache.

Complications of coeliac disease

- Lymphoma usually presents as recurrence of diarrhoea, associated with both weight loss and lassitude in a patient with established coeliac disease.
- Small bowel adenocarcinoma – presenting with non-specific symptoms, diarrheoa or constipation, weight loss, or intestinal obstruction.
- There is also an increased prevalence of carcinoma of the colon and oesophagus.
- Ulcerative jejuno-ileitis: an unusual complication associated with ulceration and stricturing.
- Microscopic colitis: a minority of patients experience concomitant colitis.

- Patients with coeliac disease have an increased prevalence of diabetes mellitus
- Infertility is common in untreated patients
- Ataxia may occur rarely
- Osteoporosis may occur in later life.

Intestinal TB

- Although this section will deal with TB affecting the intestine, the chronic infection may affect any part of the gastrointestinal system.
- Common in underdeveloped countries, certain ethnic groups (Blacks and Asians), HIV patients.
- Usually due to *Mycobacterium tuberculosis* or *M bovis*, other mycobacteria such as *M avium* and *M intracellulare* being less common.
- 25 per cent of patients with intestinal TB will also have pulmonary TB

Pathological lesions of intestinal TB

- The ileo-caecal area is reported to be the area most commonly involved in colonic tuberculosis. The apparent affinity of the tubercle bacillus for lymphoid tissue and areas of physiologic stasis facilitating prolonged contact between the bacilli and the mucosa may be the reasons for the ileum and caecum being the most common sites of disease.
- Segmental colitis involving the ascending and transverse colon
- Colonic TB may present as an inflammatory stricture
- Hypertrophic lesions resemble polyps or tumours
- Segmental ulcers and colitis
- Diffuse tuberculous colitis

Clinical presentations of intestinal TB

- Constitutional symptoms of low grade fever, sweating, weight loss
- Palpable mass especially in ileocaecal TB.
- Obstructive symptoms: pain, vomiting, weight loss and diarrhoea. Constipation is less common.
- Other manifestations are:

- Fistulae
- Mass effect
- Anaemia (iron deficiency from blood loss, vitamin B_{12} deficiency due bacterial overgrowth in stagnant bowel loops or terminal ileal involvement).
- Malabsorption

Investigations

- Bowel strictures and fistulae can be demonstrated using barium studies. Small bowel series and barium enema most often reveal a high-riding caecum with or without a string-like lesion of the terminal ileum.
- Stool cultures for TB are requested, but are very often negative.
- CT scan: tuberculous mesenteric lymphadenopathy can be difficult to distinguish from lymphoma. However, extensive infiltration of the peritoneum, omentum and mesentery – in the form of peritoneal folds thickening – and the coexistence of high-density peritoneal fluid are in favour of TB.
- Colonoscopy and biopsy.
- The diagnostic procedure of choice is colonoscopy and biopsy. Biopsies should be taken preferably from the margins of ulcerations because granulomas are often submucosal. Culture of the biopsy material may increase the diagnostic yield. However, this may give disappointing results, but polymerase chain reaction analysis of biopsy specimens obtained endoscopically has been shown to be more sensitive than culture and acid-fast stains in diagnosing intestinal TB. Indeed the quickest diagnostic method is PCR on biopsy specimens for TB nucleic acid.
- If colonoscopy is not diagnostic, laparoscopy is the next investigation that will allow visualization of the lesions and to take appropriate biopsies for histology and microbiological examination.
- Laparotomy (elective or emergency surgery for obstructive symptoms) is sometimes the only way to uncover the diagnosis.

Differential diagnosis of TB enteritis

- Crohn's disease

- Right sided colonic tumours
- Intestinal lymphoma
- *Yersinia enterocolitica*
- Amoeboma
- Gastrointestinal histoplasmosis
- Peri-appendiceal abscess

LINKS TO BOOK ONE

1. Case 38, page 118. Protein losing enteropathy.
2. Case 63, page 199. Hypogammaglobulinaemia (selective IgA deficiency and coeliac disease).

Case 47

Amoebic Liver Abscess

A 48-year-old university teacher was brought to the casualty department. Until 2 months ago, he was working for an electrical firm in Saudi Arabia. He was complaining of right-sided chest pain of five days duration. The pain was pleuritic in nature. He had no cough, haemoptysis or breathlessness. Four weeks ago while still in Saudi Arabia, he was treated by a General Practitioner for diarrhoea with loperamide. There was no history of vomiting or abdominal pain. On examination, he was pyrexial (39° Celsius) and there was a right sided pleural rub. There was marked tenderness in the right lower intercostal spaces and the right hypochondrium.

HB	14.3 g/dl
WBC	24 x 10^9/l (neutrophils 77%)
Platelets	55 x10^9/l
CXR	elevated right hemidiaphragm

What is the most likely diagnosis?

A. Streptococcal pneumonia
B. Acute empyema
C. Amoebic liver abscess
D. Sub-pulmonary pleural effusion
E. Right sided pleural effusion

Answers (C)

DISCUSSION

This patient was pyrexial with a marked leucocytosis and neutrophilia. An infective process is therefore, the most likely diagnosis such as pneumonia or liver abscess. The presence of thrombocytopenia without anaemia makes the diagnosis of a serious underlying myeloproliferative disorder less likely. Disseminated intravascular coagulation (DIC) secondary to sepsis is the most probable explanation and hence the following investigations are appropriate:

- Blood cultures
- Abdominal ultrasound: hepatic abscess or sub-phrenic collection of fluid or pus
- Arterial blood gases
- Stool examinations for *Entamoeba histolytica*
- Plasma FDP and coagulation studies to confirm DIC

The increased prevalence of amoebiasis in Saudi Arabia makes amoebic hepatitis or amoebic liver abscess the most likely diagnosis. The diagnosis of the latter is supported clinically by the exquisite tenderness in the right intercostal spaces, right hypochondrium and the raised right hemidiaphgram. Amoebiasis has to be considered in someone from the Middle East who presents with these symptoms and signs after a bout of diarrhoea.

Case 48

Gilbert's Syndrome

A 68-year-old gentleman attended the pre-operative assessment clinic prior to an inguinal hernia operation. He had no significant previous medical history. He was a non-smoker and drank two pints of beer at weekends. The biochemistry tests revealed the following:

Bilirubin	33 μmol/l
AST	20 U/l
ALT	25 U/l
ALP	52 U/l
Albumin	38 g/l

What is the most likely diagnosis?

A. Mild obstructive jaundice
B. Chronic active hepatitis B
C. Gilbert's syndrome
D. Acute hepatitis A
E. Acute alcoholic hepatitis

Answer (C)

DISCUSSION

Gilbert's Syndrome

Gilbert's syndrome is present in about 1-2 per cent of the population. The only abnormality is the mildly raised serum bilirubin, without any evidence of hepatocyte necrosis or biliary obstruction. Although it is familial, the exact mode of inheritance is not known. In Gilbert's syndrome, there is imperfect uptake and conjugation of bilirubin by the hepatocytes, resulting in mild unconjugated hyperbilirubinaemia. The serum bilirubin fluctuates and usually does not rise to levels associated with jaundice unless the patient is anorexic or has a concurrent illness. The prognosis is excellent. Liver biopsy is not justified. The following tests may be used to confirm the diagnosis:

Fasting bilirubin

Starvation increases unconjugated and conjugated serum bilirubin to twice normal levels in both healthy individuals and those with Gilbert's syndrome. However, starvation does not lead to an increase in serum bilirubin among patients with hepatocellular jaundice, haemolysis or cirrhosis.

Nicotinic acid test

Intravenous administration of nicotinic acid (50 mg) causes a rise in serum-unconjugated bilirubin among normal subjects that peaks after 90 minutes. However, in patients with Gilbert's syndrome, the rise in serum bilirubin is higher and peaks later.

LINKS TO BOOK ONE

1. Case 65, page 206. Section on liver function tests.
2. Case 67, page 219. Viral hepatitis and the viral hepatitis alphabet.

Case 49

Ulcerative Colitis Complicated by Sclerosing Cholangitis

A 53-year-old man recently arrived back in the UK from Thailand, where he had lived for the last 13 years. He developed bloody diarrhoea during the past 4 weeks with up to 5 loose motions a day, which were not associated with tenesmus or abdominal pain. The appetite was poor and he lost 4 kg in weight. On examination, he was afebrile and there was non-tender hepatomegaly to 5 cm below the costal margin in the mid-clavicular line.

Hb	9.2 g/dl
WBC	5.2×10^9/l
Platelets	432×10^9/l
ESR	44 mm/h
Na	130 mmol/l
K	3.2 mmol/l
Urea	5.2 mmol/l
Creatinine	128 μmol/l
Bilirubin	28 μmol/l
AST	156 U/l
ALT	188 U/l
ALP	844 U/l

What is the most likely diagnosis?

A. Leptospirosis
B. Amoebic liver disease
C. Acute diverticulitis and secondary liver abscess
D. Ulcerative colitis complicated with sclerosing cholangitis
E. Traveller's diarrhoea

Answer (D)

Discussion

Although amoebiasis has yet to be excluded, the *non-tender* hepatomegaly makes this diagnosis and that of bacterial liver abscess unlikely. Stool samples should be examined for *Entamoeba histolytica* and other dysenteric organisms. The markedly raised ALP is compatible with cholestasis or hepatic infiltration. The history of bloody diarrhoea and elevated ESR suggest inflammatory bowel disease, such as ulcerative colitis, which can be complicated by sclerosing cholangitis. The most important investigations are sigmoidoscopy, rectal biopsy and abdominal ultrasound. The diagnosis of sclerosing cholangitis can be established by endoscopic retrograde cholangiopancreatography.

Causes of intrahepatic cholestasis

- Infection: viral hepatitis, bacterial infections such as sepsis and leptospirosis
- Immune: chronic active hepatitis
- Drug induced hepatitis
- Infiltration: such as metastastic carcinoma, lymphoma and sarcoidosis
- Toxins
- Alcohol
- Contraceptive pill (estrogen)
- Primary biliary cirrhosis
- Sclerosing cholangitis
- Pregnancy

Causes of extrahepatic cholestasis

- Gall stones in common bile duct
- Cancer of the biliary tree
- Cancer of the pancreas
- Periampullary carcinoma
- Benign biliary strictures
- Acute pancreatitis with pseudocyst

Drug induced jaundice

Some examples of how drugs may cause jaundice are given below:

Cholestatic jaundice	1. Phenothiazine 2. Sex hormones 3. Dextropropoxyphene 4. Cimetidine and ranitidine 5. Oral hypoglycaemic agents i.e. chlorpropamide 6. Erythromycin 7. Nitrofurantoin 8. Azathioprine 9. Ciclosporin
Acute hepatitis	1. Paracetamol overdose 2. Isoniazid 3. Rifampicin 4. Cytotoxic drugs 5. Niacin 6. Halothane
Chronic hepatitis	1. Methyldopa 2. Isoniazid 3. Nitrofurantoin 4. Fenofibrate
Generalised hypersensitivity	1. Sulfonamides 2. Penicillins 3. NSAID 4. Diltiazem 5. Phenytoin 6. Carbimazole and propylthiouracil

Extra-colonic manifestations of ulcerative colitis

The extra-colonic manifestations may be related or unrelated to the activity of the colonic disease. If related to disease activity they undergo remission on treating the colitis.

- Skin and mucosal lesions. Erythema nodosum and pyoderma gangrenosum are seen in 1-2 per cent of patients along with aphthous ulcers. Skin lesions regress with treatment of colitis.
- Eye involvement. Episcleritis or uveitis is seen in about 5 per cent of patients. These resolve with local steroids and treating active colitis.
- Joint disease. Arthritis is seen in 10 to 15 per cent of patients and usually symmetrical (e.g. wrists, elbows, hips, knees, ankles). Sacroiliitis and ankylosing spondylitis are more common in colitic patients who possess the HLA-B27 antigen.

- Liver disease. Patients may have mild elevations of liver enzymes, which return to normal once remission is achieved. In addition sclerosing cholangitis can develop and lead to portal hypertension, liver failure and cholangiocarcinoma.

The following features are related to disease activity

- Aphthous ulceration of the mouth
- Erythema nodosum
- Pyoderma gangrenosum
- Episcleritis
- Uveitis
- Peripheral arthropathy
- Fatty liver

LINKS TO BOOK ONE

1. Case 55, page 169. Crohn's disease.
2. Case 89, page 302. Primary biliary cirrhosis.

Case 50

Whipple's Disease

A 56-year-old man was referred by his General Practitioner for investigation of diarrhoea and weight loss. He had been suffering from loose motions for the last 2 months with the bowels opening three to four times a day. There was no bleeding or tenesmus. He also had vague central abdominal pain, which was not related to food or bowel action. He denied vomiting or fever. The General practitioner had prescribed rofecoxib for mild joint pains involving the knees, left shoulder and left wrist. He had lost 10 kg in weight despite a normal appetite. On examination, he was rather pigmented with a few tender lymph nodes in the neck and left axilla. There was no finger clubbing or hepatosplenomegaly. Rectal examination was normal.

Hb	12.6 g/dl
WBC	7.2×10^9/l
Platelets	342×10^9/l
ESR	100 mm/h
Na	138 mmol/l
K	3.2 mmol/l
Urea	2.8 mmol/l
Creatinine	98 μmol/l
Bilirubin	18 μmol/l
ALT	32 U/l
ALP	136 U/l
Albumin	28 g/l
Total protein	71 g/l
TSH	3.8 mU/l
Stool cultures	negative
Stool parasites	negative

Flexible sigmoidoscopy	normal
Barium enema	normal
Rheumatoid factor	negative
ANA	negative
Coeliac disease antibodies	negative
Jejunal biopsy	lamina propria infiltrated with macrophages containing PAS positive deposits.

What is the most likely diagnosis?

A. Whipple's disease
B. Crohn's disease of the small bowel
C. Intestinal lymphoma
D. Behçet's syndrome
E. Tuberculous enteritis

Answer (A)

DISCUSSION

Whipple's Disease

Whipple's disease is an infectious disease caused by a rod-shaped bacterium (*Tropheryma whippelii*). It is a rare multi-system disease and occurs predominantly in males aged 30 to 60 years.

Clinical features

1. Gastrointestinal manifestations
   - Chronic diarrhoea
   - Malabsorption with steatorrhoea and protein losing enteropathy
2. Extra-intestinal features
   - Central nervous system (seizures, dementia, ophthalmoplegia)
   - Cardiac (valvular regurgitation, heart failure)
   - Arthritis (migratory involvement of large joints)
   - Peripheral lymphadenopathy
   - Ocular (uveitis, retinitis)
3. Systemic manifestations
   - Fever
   - Loss of appetite
   - Weight loss

- Increased skin pigmentation on sun-exposed areas

Investigations

1. Histology of duodenal or jejunal biopsies
   - Mucosal injury characterized by oedema and alterations in villous structure
   - Accumulation of glycoprotein-filled (PAS-positive) macrophages within the lamina propria
   - The presence of Whipple bacilli in the mucosa
2. Identification by polymerase chain reaction of the Whipple organism in biopsy material, CSF or synovial fluid
3. Investigations for malabsorption
   - Decreased D-xylose absorption
   - Anaemia (commonly due to iron deficiency, sometimes vitamin B_{12} deficiency)

Management

1. Antibiotics – various regimes are followed and it is impossible to firmly recommend any particular one. Treatment is usually for a prolonged period, may be for at least 1 year. Suggested antibiotic regimes include:
   - Trimethoprim-sulfamethoxazole
   - Penicillin and tetracycline
   - Third-generation cefalosporin
2. Supportive treatment is required until absorptive function returns to normal.
   - Fluid and electrolyte replacement
   - Iron or folate in anaemic patients
   - Vitamin D, calcium and mineral supplements as required

Case 51

Strongyloidosis

A 55-year-old tourist from Thailand presented with diarrhoea and abdominal pain of 4 weeks duration. His symptoms were mild, but became more troublesome one week after arriving in London. A private General Practitioner arranged the following investigations:

Hb	9.2 g/dl
WBC	15.2 x 10^9/l
MCV	67 fl
Neutrophils	60%
Lymphocyte	26%
Eosinophil	9%
Basophil	1%
Platelets	247 x 10^9/l
Bilirubin	18 µmol/l
ALT	28 U/l
ALP	130 U/l
Albumin	28 g/l
Total protein	60 g/l
Na	138 mmol/l
K	3.3 mmol/l
Urea	9.6 mmol/L
Creatinine	164 µmol/l
Glucose	5.2 mmol/l
Stool cultures (3 samples)	negative
CXR	normal

The patient was reassured and given advice to take plenty of fluids and loperamide as required. His symptoms persisted and he was referred to a private consultant physician. It transpired that three months ago the patient had a febrile illness with cough and an itchy rash over the legs. His FBC was repeated and showed:

Hb	9.0 g/dl
WBC	16 x 10^9/l
Neutrophils	61%
Lymphocyte	24%
Eosinophil	11%
Monocyte	4%
Platelets	381 x 10^9/l

Sigmoidoscopy showed no mass and the colonic mucosa was normal. Stool cultures were repeated and examined for parasites. The diagnosis was finally established.

What is the most likely diagnosis?

A. *Entamoeba histolytica*
B. *Giardia lamblia*
C. *Taenia saginata*
D. *Strongyloidosis*
E. *Enterobius vermicularis*

Answer (D)

DISCUSSION

Strongyloides stercoralis

Strongyloides stercoralis is an intestinal nematode found mainly in the warm wet regions of the world such as Central America and South East Asia. The worm infects the small bowel without causing significant damage. However, heavy infestation leads to abdominal pain, diarrhoea, anaemia, hypoproteinaemia and malabsorption. Fatal systemic infection can occur in immunocompromised individuals.

The adult worms lay eggs that are passed as rhabditiform larvae. Usually the rhabditiform larvae developed into filiform larvae in the soil and these can penetrate the skin to start the human infestation again. The site of skin entry is followed by a local reaction in the form of itching, oedema, redness and urticaria. Multiple skin penetrations will lead to many focal skin lesions but these disappear within a few days. The filiform larvae migrate via the circulation to the lungs where they enter the alveoli and upper respiratory tract and then gain access to the gastrointestinal tract.

The diagnosis is established by finding the rhabditiform larvae in the stools or duodenal aspirate. In severe infestations eosinophilia is an important feature. Therapeutic agents of benefit are thiabendazole, albendazole and ivermectin. Very rarely this condition may present in veterans who were former prisoners in Burma or Thailand during the Second World War.

Summary of intestinal nematodes

Organisms	*Site*	*Clinical features*
Enterobius vermicularis (threadworm)	Large intestine	Asymptomatic or pruritus ani
Trichuris trichiura (whipworm)	Large intestine	Usually asymptomatic but may cause colitis or rectal prolapse
Ascaris lumbricoides (roundworm)	Small intestine	Bowel obstruction, migration to appendix (appendicitis), migration to biliary tree (cholangitis). Its role in malnutrition in children is unclear.
Capillaria philippinensis	Small intestine	Malabsorption
Ankylostoma duodenale and Necator americanus (hookworm)	Small intestine	Iron deficiency anaemia

Eosinophilia

Eosinophils are leucocytes with cytoplasmic granules that stain bright red with eosin. They are larger than neutrophils and each nucleus contain two nuclei. They have an important role in allergic disorders, helminthic and protozoal diseases. Eosinophilia is said to be present if the count in the peripheral blood is $> 0.4 \times 10^9/l$. Causes of eosinophilia include:

- Allergic diseases – allergic drug reaction, hay fever, etc.
- Malignant conditions – Hodgkin's lymphoma, eosinophilic leukaemia
- Respiratory – bronchial asthma, tropical pulmonary eosinophilia, allergic bronchopulmonary apergillosis, Churg-Strauss syndrome
- Skin disease – urticaria, pemphigus, eczema
- Others – eosinophilic gastroenteritis, hypereosinophilic syndrome, sarcoidosis, hypoadrenalism.

Case 52

Pseudomembranous Colitis

An 82-year-old lady was admitted to an acute medical ward with sudden onset left iliac fossa pain, which was intermittently colicky and associated with nausea, but not vomiting. She had opened her bowels regularly in the last three days. She was known to be hypertensive. Five years ago, she had investigations for rectal bleeding and constipation. Diverticular disease was confirmed with barium enema and colonoscopy. Her only medications were colofac 135 mg tds and bendroflumethiazide 2.5 mg od. On examination, she was mildly pyrexial at 37.8° Celsius, the heart rate was regular at 110 bpm and blood pressure 138/72 mm Hg. The chest was clear. There was tenderness in the left iliac fossa without peritonism. Rectal examination was normal. The chest X-ray showed no free gas under the diaphragms. The abdominal X-ray did not show fluid levels or distended bowel loops.

Hb	13.2 g/dl
WBC	14.2 x 10^9/l
Platelets	347 x 10^9/l
CRP	250 mg/l
Na	144 mmol/l
K	3.2 mmol/l
Urea	11.2 mmol/l
Creatinine	142 μmol/l

A provisional diagnosis of acute diverticulitis was made. She was treated with rehydration and intravenous cefuroxime and metronidazole. Her symptoms settled over the next three days. The following week she developed watery diarrhoea 3 to 4 times each day without blood loss. Stool samples were positive for *Clostridium difficile* toxin. The patient was barrier nursed.

What is the next most appropriate management?

A. Switch the existing antibiotic (cefuroxime and metronidazole) to ciprofloxacin
B. Arrange urgent sigmoidoscopy and biopsy
C. Stop cefuroxime and metronidazole and commence the patient on oral vancomycin
D. Prescribe codeine phosphate orally to stop the diarrhoea
E. Prescribe intravenous methyl prednisolone 1 gram daily for three days

Answer (C)

DISCUSSION

Antibiotic Associated Colitis

Antibiotic associated colitis (or pseudomembranous colitis) is due to *Clostridium difficile.*

- *C difficile* is a gram positive, spore forming, anaerobic bacillus. The spores can survive for several months in the environment.
- *C difficile* can be isolated in 3 to 5 per cent of healthy adults and asymptomatic colonization is much commoner in the elderly. The presence of IgG antibody against clostridial toxin A may prevent the clinical expression of disease.
- *C difficile* colitis occurs in 20 per cent of hospitalised patients who are taking antibiotics; possibly twice these numbers are asymptomatic carriers.
- Any antibiotic can cause *C difficile* colitis, but the most common culprits are amoxicillin, ampicillin, cefalosporins, and clindamycin. Even metronidazole and vancomycin have been implicated.
- Elimination of the normal protective bowel bacteria by antibiotic therapy allows *C difficile* to proliferate and colonize the gut. *C difficile* colitis without prior antibiotic exposure can occur in patients with pre-existing bowel disease, uraemia, cancer and following antineoplastic chemotherapy.
- The *C difficile* bacterium produces two cytotoxins, toxin A and B, which bind to intestinal receptors, leading ultimately to disruption of the cellular cytoskeleton and intracellular junctions.
- The term pseudomembranous colitis is derived from the macroscopic appearance of yellow inflammatory plaques that are found adherent to the colonic mucosa.

- *C difficile* colitis is more common in older hospitalised patients. The onset of symptoms usually occurs within 2 weeks of antibiotic treatment, but may be delayed for several weeks. Symptoms include diarrhoea, often with mucus and blood, cramp-like abdominal pain, and fever. Severe cases can develop toxic megacolon. Prolonged diarrhoea may be complicated by hypoalbuminaemia and wasting.

Diagnostic tests for C difficile

- Diagnosis is based on demonstrating *C difficile* toxins in stool specimens. Only diarrhoeal stool should be tested, as asymptomatic carriage is common. Identification of the organism from stool culture is difficult and does not distinguish between toxin producing strains from non-toxin producing ones. Plain X-rays or CT may show oedema of the bowel wall, which is descriptively called "thumb printing", but this finding is not specific and can occur in any form of bowel inflammation. Sigmoidoscopic examination is unnecessary in antibiotic associated colitis and may have a higher risk of colonic perforation in sick patients.
- Enzyme linked immunosorbent assays (ELISA) can detect 100 to 1000 pg of toxin A and B, and the result is available within one day. There is a false negative rate of around 10 to 20 per cent due to low stool toxin levels. One per cent of *Clostridium difficile* strains produce only the B toxin. Therefore, it is important to check the laboratory assay is able to detect both toxins of *Clostridium difficile* and more than one stool specimen should be sent.
- Tissue culture cytotoxicity assay is very sensitive and can detect as little as 10 pg of toxin in the stool. However, tissue culture is not generally available and this method will take up to 3 days to produce a test result.
- PCR for toxin A and B is expensive and not generally available.

The differential diagnosis of antibiotic associated colitis

- *Salmonella, Shigella* and *Campylobacter gastroenteritis*
- Crohn's disease
- Ulcerative colitis

Treatment of antibiotic associated colitis

- Stop the precipitating antibiotic and allow the colitis to resolve spontaneously
- Rehydration and correction of electrolyte disturbances
- Metronidazole (400 mg tds orally for 10-14 days) or vancomycin (125 mg tds or qds orally for 10-14 days). Metronidazole is used first line as it is considerably cheaper than vancomycin. Severe cases of toxic megacolon may need IV metronidazole. IV vancomycin will be ineffective as hardly any of the drug enters the stool when given parenterally. Use oral vancomycin if there has been no response to 3 days of metronidazole. Other situations where vancomycin is preferred over metronidazole are pregnancy and in lactating women.
- Barrier nursing to confine the infection and avoid spread to other patients
- Codeine and loperamide are generally avoided

Recurrent Clostridium difficile colitis

About 20 per cent of patients will relapse following a standard course of treatment with either metronidazole or vancomycin. About 5 per cent of patients have more than 6 relapses. The therapeutic options for relapsing *Clostridium difficile* colitis are:

- Prescribe another course of metronidazole or vancomycin.
- Prolonged and tapered course of vancomycin over 6 weeks: 125 mg qds for 7 days; 125mg bd x 7 days; 125 mg od x 7 days; 125 mg every other day x 7 days; 125 mg every 3rd day x 14 days. This regime will allow clostridial spores to germinate into their vegetative forms, which then become susceptible to vancomycin and permit the normal gut flora to re-establish.
- Cholestyramine 4 g tds orally for 14 days. Cholestyramine is believed to bind to clostridial toxin and can be administered with vancomycin. As cholestyramine can bind to vancomycin and other drugs, the two agents must not be taken within 3 hours of each other.
- Vancomycin 125 mg qds and rifampicin 300 mg bd can be given orally for 14 days.
- Saccharomyces boulardii and Saccharomyces cerevisiae (Brewer's yeast) are believed to bind to clostridial toxin A or

its intestinal receptor. Both can be used in combination with either metronidazole or vancomycin.

- *Lactobacillus* GG may inhibit proliferation of *Clostridium* and increase IgA and IgG at the colonic mucosa.
- IV gammaglobulin to boost antibody immunity, as relapses are commoner in those patients with low IgG antibodies to toxin A. In future anti-toxin A antibody response may be augmented by immunization.
- Restoring normal bowel flora with rectal infusion of normal faecal organisms has been described, but may transmit other diseases.

REFERENCE

1. Mylonakis E et al. *Clostridium difficile*-associated diarrhoea. A review. Arch Intern Med 2001;161:525-33.
2. Bartlett JG. Antibiotic-associated diarrhoea. NEJM 2002;346:334-40.

LINKS TO BOOK ONE

1. Case 38, page 118. Protein losing enteropathy.
2. Case 55, page 169. Crohn's disease.

Case 53

Faecal Impaction with Overflow Diarrhoea

A 68-year-old lady was referred to the A and E department by her General Practitioner. She lived in a nursing home where she was pleasantly confused, bed bound and completely dependent for assistance in all her daily activities. Her past medical history included hypertension, multiple strokes and vascular dementia. Her regular medications were aspirin 75 mg od, 2 senna tablets nocte and nifedipine 10 mg tds. Her main problem was diarrhoea and faecal incontinence. She had been opening her bowels 4-5 times a day, passing liquid motions without blood. She had no abdominal pain but vomited twice. On examination, she was disorientated and confused, but haemodynamically stable with a blood pressure 130/70 mm Hg and a regular heart rate of 88 bpm. The abdomen was not distended and bowel sounds were present.

Hb	11.4 g/dl
WBC	6.2×10^9/l
Platelets	280×10^9/l
Bilirubin	17 μmol/l
ALT	28 U/l
ALP	120 U/l
Albumin	30 g/l
Total protein	61 g/l
Na	152 mmol/l
K	5.2 mmol/l
Urea	9.3 mmol/l
Creatinine	143 μmol/l
Corrected calcium	2.4 mmol/l
Glucose	5.2 mmol/l

CXR	normal cardiac size, no focal lung lesion, no free gas under the diaphragms.
Abdominal X-ray	no evidence of bowel obstruction

The medical SHO diagnosed infective diarrhoea, arranged stool cultures and started her on intravenous fluids. Three days later, the patient still had diarrhoea and stool cultures were negative. She also developed urinary retention and required catheterisation. The medical registrar did a rectal examination and made the definitive diagnosis.

What is the most likely diagnosis?

A. Viral gastroenteritis
B. Acute diverticulitis
C. Rectovesical fistula
D. Ulcerative colitis
E. Faecal impaction with overflow diarrhoea

Answer (E)

DISCUSSION

Faecal Impaction with Overflow Diarrhoea

This patient's problem was overlooked because rectal examination was not performed on admission. The loose stools were due to overflow faecal matter over impacted faeces. Impacted faeces also caused retention of urine. The medical registrar's examining finger discovered a large hard faecal mass sitting just above the anal verge, which required a cleansing enema. Subsequently, a barium enema showed multiple left sided colonic diverticulae.

Diverticular disease is very common in elderly and asymptomatic in 90 per cent of patients. It does not present as acute retention of urine and overflow faecal incontinence. When symptomatic, the clinical presentations include:

- Alteration of bowel habits and may be mis-diagnosed as irritable bowel syndrome
- Rectal bleeding
- Iron deficiency anaemia. It is a good practice to exclude other sinister conditions, such as tumours of the colon, as a cause of chronic blood loss before attributing it to diverticular disease.
- Acute diverticulitis

Complications of acute diverticulitis

- Bleeding
- Perforation (see figure below which shows two small paracolic abscesses) and peritonitis
- Fistulae into the vagina or bladder
- Intestinal obstruction

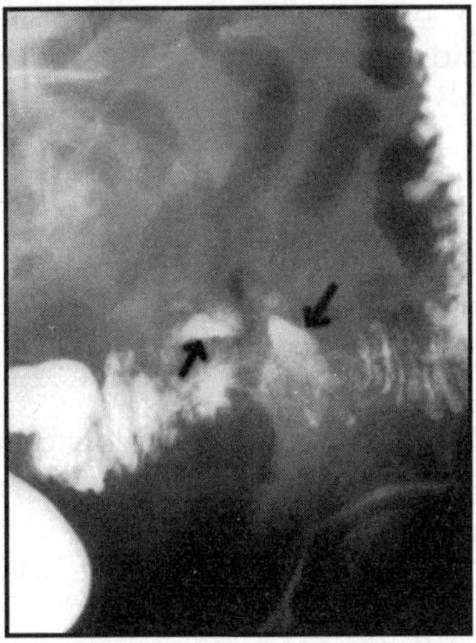

Diarrhoea

- Diarrhoea is defined as the abnormal passage of loose or liquid stools more than three times daily.
- Diarrhoea is a stool volume greater than 200 gram per day in the western world and 400 gm per day in the eastern world. In clinical practice, the volume of stool per day is seldom useful in diagnosing organic diarrhoea.

When a patient has diarrhoea the following questions should be asked:

- Is diarrhoea due to a systemic disease?
- Is this small bowel or large bowel diarrhoea?
- What is the definitive cause of the diarrhoea?
- Are there systemic complications?
- If no organic cause has been identified, is this functional diarrhoea?

The features, which suggest an organic disease are:

- Nocturnal diarrhoea

- Weight loss
- Bleeding with stools or blood stained stools with diarrhoea
- Steatorrhoea
- Symptoms > 4 weeks duration

Differentiation of small bowel disease from colonic or inflammatory forms of diarrhoea is easier if the patient has typical steatorrhoea of malabsorption. The passage of bulky malodorous pale stools indicates steatorrhoea of malabsorption. On the other hand, colonic, inflammatory or secretary forms of diarrhoea typically present with liquid loose stools with blood or mucous discharge.

Chronic diarrhoea can result from an organic or a functional bowel disturbance. The latter is more likely if there are no ALARM symptoms such as bleeding, weight loss or constitutional features. A small list of the common causes of diarrhoea should be remembered including: small bowel disease, colonic disease, systemic diseases and infections.

Causes of diarrhoea

Colonic causes

- Ulcerative and Crohn's colitis
- Recent antibiotic therapy and exclude *Clostridium difficile* infection.
- Colonic resection
- Colonic neoplasia

Small bowel disease

- Coeliac disease
- Crohn's disease
- Other: Whipple's disease, tropical sprue, amyloid, intestinal lymphangiectasia

Bile acid malabsorption

- **Disaccharidase deficiency**
- Small bowel bacterial overgrowth
- Extensive small bowel resection (reduced area for absorption) and large bowel resection
- Mesenteric ischaemia
- Radiation enteritis
- Lymphoma

Pancreatic

- **Chronic pancreatitis**
- Pancreatic carcinoma
- Cystic fibrosis

Endocrine

- **Hyperthyroidism**
- Diabetes mellitus
- Hypoparathyroidism
- Addison's disease
- Hormone secreting tumours (e.g. VIP-oma, gastrinoma, carcinoid)

Alcohol abuse

- Rapid gut transit
- Decreased activity of intestinal disaccharidases
- Decreased pancreatic function

Drugs

- Acarbose, metformin
- Magnesium salts and laxative abuse
- Antihypertensive
- Non-steroidal anti-inflammatory drugs (COX 2 inhibitors)
- Proton pump inhibitors
- Theophyllines, antibiotics
- Antiarrhythmics
- Cytotoxic drugs

Recent overseas travel (traveller's diarrhoea)

Viruses	1. Rota virus 2. Small round virus (Norwalk agent)
Bacteria	1. *Shigella* sp. 2. *Campylobacter jejuni* 3. *Vibrio cholerae* 4. *Salmonella* sp. 5. Non-cholera vibrios e.g. V. parahaemolyticus

Protozoa	1. *Giardia lamblia*
	2. *Entamoeba histolytica*
	3. *Cryptosporidium*

The investigation of diarrhoea

1. Baseline investigations such as full blood count, erythrocyte sedimentation rate, electrolytes, liver function tests, iron studies, vitamin B_{12}, folate, calcium level and thyroid function should be carried out. High erythrocyte sedimentation rate, anaemia or low albumin suggests organic disease.
2. Examination of three fresh stool specimens for ova, cysts and parasites to rule out protozoan infections, such as giardiasis and amoebiasis, which most likely result in chronic infections.
3 Further tests to investigate colonic diarrhoea should be stratified:
   - Flexible sigmoidoscopy (and biopsy if required) is the preferred investigation. However, this investigation will miss right-sided colonic lesions.
   - Colonoscopy will be required if the sigmoidoscopy did not reveal a significant pathology to explain the diarrhoea. This is especially important to diagnose or exclude right sided colonic pathological conditions such as:
     - Neoplasms and polyps
     - Crohn's disease
     - Ileocaecal TB
     - Lymphomas, etc
   - However very frail elderly people may not tolerate these investigations.
   - Barium enema. Colonoscopy is a more sensitive test than barium enema in lower gastrointestinal lesions. In addition, colonoscopy will allow tissue diagnosis. However, the barium enema provides additional information such as the detailed anatomical assessment, extent of previous colonic surgery, presence or absence of fistulae and the extent of inflammatory bowel disease.
   - Small bowel imaging (barium follow through) should be reserved for cases where small bowel malabsorption is suspected and distal duodenal histology is normal.
   - Bacterial overgrowth. In patients with small bowel bacterial overgrowth, culture of jejunal aspirates or unwashed small

bowel biopsies remains the gold standard and should be encouraged whenever this diagnosis is seriously considered.

- Empirical therapy is encouraged in patients with the diagnoses of pancreatic insufficiency, bile acid malabsorption, and small bowel bacterial overgrowth.
- ^{99m}Technetium hexa-methyl-propyleneamine oxime (Tc-HMPAO) labelled white cell scanning is a non-invasive useful technique for detecting intestinal inflammation and terminal ileal Crohn's disease.
- In some cases a definitive diagnosis is not possible. These are patients with watery, secretory, self-limiting "idiopathic" diarrhoea (presumably infective) or undiagnosed factitious diarrhoea. In the majority of these patients the prognosis is good and hence, further investigations are not warranted and symptomatic treatment should be instituted.

Factitious diarrhoea

Factitious diarrhoea is due to laxative abuse or the spurious adding of water or urine to stool specimens. Low stool volume (less than 200 ml per day) and low stool osmolality (< 290 mosmol/kg) support the diagnosis. The likelihood of this diagnosis increases if numerous and repeated investigations reveal negative results.

Case 54

Chronic GI Blood Loss

A 58-year-old man was referred for the investigation of excessive tiredness. There was no significant past medical history and he has not been on any medications. The initial blood tests showed:

Hb	8.2 g/dl
WBC	$5.8 \times 10^9/l$
Platelets	$462 \times 10^9/l$
MCV	67 fl
MCH	29 pg
Faecal occult blood	positive

His General Practitioner had organised an urgent gastroscopy, which was normal. Subsequently a barium enema showed a 2 cm polyp in the descending colon.

What is the next most appropriate step in management?

A. Referral for left hemicolectomy
B. Colonoscopy and biopsy
C. Measurement of carcinoembryonic antigen level
D. Reassurance and follow-up in 3 months
E. Diagnostic laparotomy

Answer (B)

DISCUSSION

The most common cause of hypochromic–microcytic (reduced MCV, MCH, and MCHC) anaemia is chronic iron deficiency. Other causes include:

- Chronic disorders can occasionally present with mildly hypochromic anaemia

- Sideroblastic anaemia
- Thalassaemia
- Congenital transferrin deficiency

Causes of Iron deficiency anaemia

The main causes of iron deficiency anaemia are:

- Blood loss: overt or occult. The most common causes are from the gastrointestinal tract and uterus. However, other important routes of blood loss are the urinary tract, retroperitonium and arterial tree (as in ruptured aortic aneurysm).
- Poor dietary intake.
- Malabsorption syndrome
- Increased metabolic demand such as during growth spurts (i.e. childhood) and during pregnancy

Investigation of chronic blood loss from the gastrointestinal tract

The usual scenario is a patient with iron deficiency anaemia and positive faecal occult bloods. In the absence of definite clues to an upper or lower digestive tract condition, it is generally preferable to start at the top end. Consequently, the following investigations are arranged in the order listed:

- Gastroscopy with duodenal biopsy (if indicated)
- Sigmoidoscopy
- Barium enema
- Colonoscopy

Case 55

Chronic Hepatitis B Virus Carrier State

A 44-year-old teacher from India presented with right upper quadrant abdominal pain. There was no history of jaundice or drug abuse. She did not smoke but took one glass of wine each day. She was concerned about viral hepatitis.

Bilirubin	28 µmol/l
ALT	38 U/l
ALP	116 U/l
Albumin	41 g/l
HAV IgG	negative
HBsAg	positive
HBeAg	negative
Anti-HBe antibody	positive
HBV-DNA	negative

What is the most likely diagnosis?

A. Acute viral hepatitis A
B. Acute viral hepatitis B
C. Chronic hepatitis B
D. Hepatitis C virus infection
E. Chronic hepatitis B virus carrier state

Answer (E)

DISCUSSION

The clinical outcomes of acute HBV infection

- Acute hepatitis: 25 per cent (recovery = 99%, mortality =1%)
- Transient sub-clinical infection: 65 per cent (recovery = 100%)
- Chronic HBV infection: 10 per cent

- Healthy HBsAg carrier: 70-90 per cent (possible cause of hepatocellular carcinoma).
- Chronic hepatitis 10-30 per cent. This may be complicated by cirrhosis or carcinoma of the liver.

Chronic carrier of HBV

- HBsAg positive
- HBeAg negative
- Anti-HBe antibody positive
- HBV DNA blood negative
- No evidence of liver disease
- Not likely infectious
- Does not develop active liver disease
- Annual clearance rate 1 to 2 per cent

Note: Individuals who have HBeAg and HBV DNA in their serum are not true carriers, but have an occult liver disease.

The clinical significance of HBV antibodies

Antigens	*Clinical significance*
HBsAg	1. Acute or chronic infection 2. Appears and stays for about 6 weeks to 3 months and then disappears
HBeAg	1. It is present in acute hepatitis B 2. Appears after HBsAg and declines in < 3 months 3. Its persistence may indicate: • continuous infectious state • development of chronicity • increased severity of disease
HBV-DNA	1. Viral replication

The clinical significance of HBV antibodies

Antibodies		*Clinical significance*
Anti-HBs		• Immunity to HBV (previous exposure) • Appears late and indicates immunity
Anti-HBe		• Indicates seroconversion • Indicates decreased infectivity i.e. low risk • Appears after HBc antibody
Anti-HBc	IgM high titres	• Acute hepatitis
	IgM low titres	• Chronic hepatitis
	IgG	• Past exposure to HBV (HBsAg negative)

Prophylaxis against Hepatitis B viral infection

- Avoidance of exposure
- Active immunization
- Passive immunization

Avoidance of exposure

In the developing countries, unnecessary exposure may be still encountered by blood transfusion and use of blood products. Non-disposable syringes are used in some parts of the world with poverty stricken health services. The following are important sources of HBV transmission all over the world:

- Shared needles
- Homosexual males with multiple partners
- Prostitution

Individuals with HBV DNA and HBeAg in their serum or liver have high infectivity.

Active immunization

Hepatitis B vaccine is a recombinant vaccine produced by insertion of a plasmid containing the HBsAg gene into yeast. It should be given to the following groups:

- All health care personnel
- Members of the rescue and emergency services
- Morticians and embalmers
- People with high risk life style: homosexuals, bisexuals, IV drug abusers, prostitutes
- Haemophiliacs
- Children from high risk areas
- Long term travellers
- Sexual partners of HBV positive patients
- Patients in some psychiatric units (discuss with public health services)

Combined prophylaxis (vaccination and passive immunization with immunoglobulins)

The indications for the combined prophylaxis are:

- Health care staff with accidental needle stick injury.
- All babies born to mothers who are HBsAg positive.

- Regular sexual partners of HBsAg positive patients, who have been found to be HBVnegative

The doses of specific Hepatitis B immunoglobulin (HBIG) for passive immunization are:

- Adults 500 IU
- Children 200 IU

It is important that the HBIG and vaccine are given at different sites.

LINKS TO BOOK ONE

1. Case 67, page 219. Viral hepatitis and the viral hepatitis alphabet.

Case 56

Pulmonary Stenosis

A 28-year-old man has a systolic murmur at the left sternal edge. The cardiac catheter data showed:

RA pressure	5/0 mmHg
RV pressure	70/6 mmHg
Main pulmonary artery pressure	30/15 mmHg

Oxygen saturation studies showed:

SVC	75%
RA	74%
RV	74%
PA	72%

What is the diagnosis?

A. Pulmonary stenosis
B. Atrial septal defect
C. Patent foramen ovale
D. Tricuspid stenosis
E. Right ventricular dysplasia

Answer (A)

DISCUSSION

Pulmonary Stenosis

The normal right-sided pressures are as follows:

RA	0-5 mmHg
RV	18-30 mmHg (systolic); 0-5 mmHg (diastolic)
PA	18-30 mmHg (systolic); 6-12 mmHg (diastolic)
PCWP	6-12 mmHg
LA	4-8 mmHg

The higher systolic right ventricular pressure compared to the systolic pulmonary artery pressure indicates obstruction at the level of the right ventricular outflow tract i.e. pulmonary stenosis. An echocardiogram showed diffuse right ventricular hypertrophy. There is no step up of oxygen saturation at the right side, which means there is no reversed shunt.

Case 57

Absent 'a' Wave

A 79-year-old man has been breathlessness for six months with bilateral ankle swelling. While lying semi-recumbent at the 45 degrees position, the top level of the internal jugular pulsation was 8 cm above the sternal angle. The heart rate was irregular at 120 bpm and blood pressure was 117/72 mm Hg. There was a pansystolic murmur at the apex radiating to the axilla. There were bibasal crepitations. The ECG showed atrial fibrillation with ST changes and T wave inversion in the anterolateral leads. The echocardiography showed poor overall systolic function with anteroseptal akinesia and a dilated left atrium. There was severe mitral and tricuspid regurgitation.

Which feature in the jugular venous pulsation suggests atrial fibrillation?

A. Prominent 'a' wave
B. Absent 'a' wave
C. Prominent 'v' wave
D. Canon waves
E. Engorged non-pulsatile internal jugular pulsation

Answer (B)

DISCUSSION

The 'a' wave in the JVP

There are no valvular structures between the internal jugular vein and the superior vena cava, and between the latter and the right atrium. Under normal circumstances, the height of the JVP is just below the clavicle. The 'a' and 'v' waves may be just visible at the clavicle. Many medical students and even doctors have difficulty in assessing the jugular venous pressure (JVP) and jugular venous pulsations. Traditionally, the height of the JVP is assessed while the patient is semi-recumbent at 30 to 45 degrees. The height of the JVP is the vertical distance between the sternal angle and the highest level of the visible internal jugular venous pulsation. These anatomical landmarks can be marked out using a ruler to indicate the level of the sternal angle and a tongue depressor for the level of jugular venous pulsation. When the JVP is markedly raised, the upper level of pulsation may not be seen in the supine patient, because it is either behind the ear or intracranial. In this situation the examiner should ask the patient to sit into the 45 degree position and if necessary lean progressively further forwards. Repositioning the patient in this way will allow the JVP to fall and become visible in the neck.

The internal jugular vein lies in the carotid sheath, which may make it difficult to be differentiated from carotid pulsations. However, the following tips are useful:

- Venous pulsations vary with respiration – falling with inspiration due to negative intrathoracic pressure.
- Gentle pressure at the base of neck abolishes the venous pulsation, but has no effect on carotid pulsations.
- Venous pressure is amplified by gentle pressure on the abdomen (hepatojugular reflux)
- Normally the jugular pulsation is wavy showing 'a' waves before the carotid pulsations while the 'v'wave follows carotid pulsation.

a = atrial contraction (during diastole).

x = this descent follows the '*a*' wave and is probably associated with the descent of the base of the heart during the ventricular systole which makes the atrio-ventricular valves (mitral and tricuspid) move towards the apex. The '*x*' descent is interrupted by the *c* wave (which is normally not visible but recordable by jugular phlebography). The '*c*' wave represents the closure of the tricuspid valve.

v = coincides with ventricular systole.

y descent = falling of the right atrial pressure when the tricuspid valve opens at onset of diastole.

Causes of raised JVP

- Right sided cardiac failure
- Fluid overload
- Acute nephritic syndrome
- Acute right ventricular infarction

Some abnormalities of jugular venous pulsations

- Absent *'a'* wave in atrial fibrillation
- Prominent *'a'* wave in tricuspid stenosis and pulmonary hypertension
- Prominent *'v'*wave in tricuspid regurgitation
- Canon waves in ventricular tachycardia.

Case 58

Pulmonary Stenosis and ASD with Left to Right Shunt

An 18-year-old man has a systolic murmur at the base of the heart.

Right heart catheter studies showed:

RA pressure	6/0 mmHg
RV pressure	60/4 mmHg
Main pulmonary artery pressure	20/10 mmHg

Oxygen saturation studies showed:

SVC	70%
RA	85%
RV	82%
PA	81%

What is the diagnosis?

A. Pulmonary stenosis
B. Atrial septal defect
C. Ventricular septal defect
D. Idiopathic pulmonary hypertension
E. Pulmonary stenosis and atrial septal defect with left to right shunt

Answer (E)

DISCUSSION

The two important findings here are:

1. The systolic right ventricular pressure is higher than the systolic pulmonary artery pressure. This indicates obstruction at the right ventricular outflow tract, such pulmonary stenosis.

2. The sudden rise in oxygen saturation in the right atrium indicates a left to right shunt at the level of the atria, i.e. atrial septal defect.

An echocardiogram showed diffuse right ventricular hypertrophy and atrial septal defect. The doppler studies confirmed the left to right shunt across the atrial septal defect.

Case 59

Aortic Dissection

A normally healthy 75-year woman collapsed while shopping. She was a known hypertensive for the last five years and was on amlodipine 5 mg od and aspirin 75 mg od. She was brought semi-conscious to the A and E department. The blood pressure was 180/110 mm Hg in the right arm and 80/40 mm Hg in the left arm. She was in atrial fibrillation with an apex heart rate of 120 bpm. There was a systolic murmur at the apex and an early diastolic murmur at the left sternal edge. The chest was clear. There was a right hemiparesis with an extensor plantar response. The ECG showed an acute inferior MI with 2-3 mm of ST segment elevation in leads V1-V6. An urgent CT brain was arranged to ascertain if there was any contraindication to thrombolysis. The result was normal. The medical registrar reviewed the patient and asked for a chest X-ray that showed a widened aortic root.

What is the most likely diagnosis?

A. Acute myocardial infarction with embolisation to left arm
B. Aortic root aneurysm
C. Aortic dissection
D. Acute pericarditis
E. Acute cerebral infarction and embolism to left subclavian artery

Answer (C)

DISCUSSION

Aortic Dissection

Dissection is a tear in the inner lining of the arterial wall and usually leads to bleeding into the vessel wall. Dissecting aortic aneurysm describes dissection that is accompanied by ballooning of the wall of the aorta. Dissection can start anywhere in the aorta, but the most common sites are the ascending aorta and the aorta distal to the left subclavian artery.

Classification

The commonest classifications used are:

A. The DeBakey Classification
   a. Type I involves the ascending aorta, aortic arch, and descending aorta.
   b. Type II is confined to the ascending aorta.
   c. Type III is confined to the descending aorta distal to the left subclavian artery and this has two subtypes:
      - Type IIIa refers to dissections that originate distal to the left subclavian artery, but extend both proximally and distally.
      - Type IIIb refers to dissections that originate distal to the left subclavian artery, extend only distally.

B. The Stanford Classification is as follows:
   a. Type A involves the ascending aorta (DeBakey types I and II) – mostly requiring surgery.
   b. Type B does not involve ascending aorta (DeBakey type III) – mostly managed medically.

Aetiology

The non-traumatic conditions associated with aortic dissection are:

- Hypertension
- Atherosclerosis
- Coarctation of aorta
- Valvular regurgitation
- Collagen disorders, including:
  - Pseudoxanthoma elasticum
  - Ehlers-Danlos syndrome
  - Marfan's syndrome
  - Relapsing polychondritis
- Syphilitic aortitis
- Cocaine use causes a rapid rise in blood pressure, which may cause aortic dissection.

Clinical features

Chest pain is the cardinal symptom, but is absent in up to 10 per cent of the patients. The pain is of abrupt onset, ripping or tearing in nature, and most severe at the onset. It may travel under the shoulder blades and radiate to the neck, jaw, arm, shoulder, abdomen and hips. Acute chest pain that escalates despite analgesia should raise the suspicion of aortic dissection. The other presentations include:

- Fainting (syncope)
- Profuse sweating
- Stroke
- Acute myocardial infarction
- Acute left ventricular failure
- Cardiogenic shock
- Cardiac tamponade
- Acute aortic regurgitation
- Ischaemia and infarction in the territory of aortic branches involved by dissection, such as arm, brain, bowel, kidney, etc.

The useful signs one should be looked for are:

- Unequal pulses in the arms
- Unequal blood pressure in the arms
- Delay in the timing of radial and femoral pulses
- Acute aortic regurgitation

Investigations

- ECG: ST-T segment changes may be seen or acute myocardial infarction (with or without Q waves)
- CXR - mediastinal widening or pleural effusion
- Transoesophageal echocardiogram (TOE) is the best diagnostic test for aortic dissection, particularly if it involves the ascending aorta where surgery is urgently needed. TOE can also provide information on the aortic valve, pericardial fluid (blood) accumulation and left ventricular function.
- MRI – shows the site of intimal tear, extent of the dissection and presence of aortic insufficiency. It has a very high specificity for the diagnosis of aortic dissection, but may not be available out of normal working hours.

- CT scan with contrast. If local expertise for transoesophageal echocardiography is not available, CT scan of the chest with contrast is the next investigation of choice particularly in district general hospitals. It will show a double lumen and aneurysmal dilatation of the aorta.
- Contrast angiography is performed under heavy sedation or general anaesthesia prior to operative treatment. It will also allow coronary angiography. Separate aortic root and aortic arch angiograms are essential and the radiocontrast is followed into the descending aorta.

Treatment

- Analgesia
- Anti-hypertensive therapy: beta-blockers to reduce the myocardial contractility and workload. The aim is to reduce the systolic blood pressure to less than 120 mm Hg and mean aortic pressure to less than 90 mm Hg. Nitroprusside is ideal because of its short half-life.
- Open-heart surgery is indicated for dissection involving the aortic root and aortic arch unless surgical intervention is considered to be futile. Patients with aortic dissection involving only the descending aorta are treated medically or surgically depending on the extent of the lesion and whether vital organs are in danger of ischaemia. Ischaemic legs indicate surgical intervention.

Prognosis

Death within 24 hours occurs in about 33 per cent of patients without surgical treatment. The mortality rate increases to 50 per cent within 48 hours and 75 per cent within two weeks of onset. The survival rate for individuals undergoing elective surgery is greater than 95 per cent. Survival rates are lower for emergency operations.

LINKS TO BOOK ONE

1. Case 88, page 298. Carotid artery dissection.

Case 60

Endocarditis and Q Fever

A 44-year-old farmer was referred with a 3 months history of shortness of breath. In the last three months, he has been suffering from aches and pains with low-grade fever, which he treated with paracetamol and ibuprofen obtained from over the counter at his local chemist. In the last two weeks, he had become more breathless and lying down aggravated his symptoms. On examination, his temperature was 38.2° Celsius, the heart rate was regular at 118 bpm and blood pressure 130/40 mmHg. In the chest, there were bilateral basal crackles and scattered wheezes.

Hb	13.2 g/dl
WBC	$7.0 \times 10^9/l$
Platelets	$172 \times 10^9/l$
Na	128 mmol/l
K	4.2 mmol/l
Urea	9 mmol/l
Creatinine	141 µmol/l
Glucose	5.3 mmol/l
Neutrophil	60%
Lymphocyte	30%
Basophil	1%
Monocyte	5%
Eosinophil	4%
CXR	patchy opacities in the left lower and right middle zones.

The medical registrar obtained blood cultures and started him on intravenous fluids amoxicillin and clarithromycin. Three days later, he continued to be pyrexial and blood cultures were still negative. He added intravenous fluids and flucloxacillin to cover for *Staphylococcus aureus*. A second set of blood cultures was taken, which came back negative 2 days later. The cardiologist detected a systolic murmur and end diastolic murmur at the left sternal edge. Echocardiography confirmed aortic regurgitation and vegetations.

What is the most likely microorganism?

A. *Mycoplasma*
B. Coxsackie B
C. *Candida albicans*
D. *Coxiella burnetii*
E. *Aspergillus fumigatus*

Answer (D)

DISCUSSION

Blood Culture in Infective Endocarditis

At least six sets of blood cultures should be taken in suspected endocarditis. Further cultures are obtained at peaks of temperature. If there is a central venous line catheter, it should be removed and the tip sent for culture. Approximately 20 per cent of patients with bacterial endocarditis have negative cultures. The most common causes of culture negative endocarditis are:

- Prior antibiotic therapy
- Bacterial infection, but late presentation and inaccessible bacteria

Infective Causes of Endocarditis:

The commonest bacteria involved are:

- The *Streptococcus viridans* group probably accounts for 50 per cent of cases and include:
  - *Streptococcus milleri*
  - *Streptococcus mutans*
  - *Streptococcus mitis*
  - *Streptococcus mitior*
- *Staphylococcus aureus* and *Staphylococcus epidermidis* together account for another 25 per cent of cases.
- The *Enterococcus* group cause approximately 10 per cent of cases.

- Other organisms include *Haemophilus influenzae, Listeria monocytogenes*, Microaerophilic streptococci, *Candida albicans, Brucella abortus*, Diphtheroid bacilli, etc.

Blood Culture Negative Endocarditis

If blood cultures are repeatedly negative, consider the following diagnoses:

- Q fever
- Aspergillosis
- Brucellosis
- *Candida albicans*
- Marantic endocarditis

Q fever

In the United States Q fever became a notifiable disease in 1999, but reporting is not required in many other countries. In England and Wales Q fever is not notifiable under the Public Health Control of Diseases Act 1984, but doctors must report certain diseases they believe to be occupationally acquired, such as Q fever, to their patient's employer. In turn, employers must report cases of these diseases to the Health and Safety Executive (HSE) under the Reporting of Injuries, Diseases and Dangerous Occurrences Regulations (RIDDOR) 1986.

Q fever is a zoonotic disease caused by *Coxiella burnetii,* which primarily infects cattle, sheep and goats. Domesticated pets may occasionally become infected. *Coxiella burnetii* does not usually cause clinical disease in animals. The organism is excreted in the milk, urine and faeces of infected animals. The most important method of transmission is the shedding of this organism with the amniotic fluid and placenta of infected animals. *Coxiella burnetii* is resistant to heat, drying and many common disinfectants, which therefore, enables the bacterium to survive for prolonged periods in the environment. Human infection occurs by inhalation of this organism from air that contains airborne barnyard dust contaminated with dried placental material, birth fluids and excreta of infected herd animals. Only a few organisms may be required to cause infection in humans. Other routes of human infection include ingestion of contaminated milk and tick bites.

Signs and symptoms of acute Q fever

The incubation period depends on the infecting dose of organisms. Infection with greater numbers of organisms will result in shorter incubation periods. Most patients become ill within 2-3 weeks after exposure. Subclinical infection is common. When symptomatic, the presentations include the following:

- Febrile illness of sudden onset with generalised malaise, myalgia, confusion, sore throat, chills and sweats. Fever usually lasts for 1 to 2 weeks.
- Respiratory illness with non-productive cough, chest pain, pneumonia.
- Gastrointestinal symptoms such as nausea, vomiting, diarrhoea, abdominal pain and weight loss.
- Abnormal liver function tests due to granulomatous hepatitis.

Only 1 to 2 per cent of people with acute Q fever die of the disease. Survivors of the acute infection may possess lifelong immunity against re-infection.

Chronic Q fever

Chronic Q fever is uncommon and may develop between 1 and 20 years after acute infection. Patients with compromised immunity (e.g. transplant recipients, cancer, and chronic kidney disease) are at risk. The mortality rate is high: 65 per cent of patients with chronic Q fever die of the disease. The most serious complication of chronic Q fever is endocarditis, usually of the aortic or mitral valves and most patients have pre-existing valvular disease or a vascular graft.

Diagnosis of Q fever

The diagnosis of Q fever can be confirmed serologically. The indirect immunofluorescence assay (IFA) is the most dependable and widely used method for detecting antibodies to *Coxiella burnetii. Coxiella burnetii* exists in two antigenic forms called phase I and phase II. In acute Q fever the antibody level to phase II is higher than to phase I. In chronic Q fever, the reverse situation is true. Therefore, high levels of phase I antibody with constant or falling levels of phase II antibody suggest chronic Q fever.

- Increased IgM levels indicate recent infection.
- Acute Q fever is suggested by IgG antibody to phase II and IgM antibody to phases I and II.

- Q fever endocarditis is indicated by increased IgG and IgA antibody levels.
- The bacterium can be identified in infected tissues using immunohistochemical staining and DNA detection methods.

Treatment of acute Q fever

- Doxycycline is the treatment of choice for acute Q fever (e.g. 100 mg bd for 15-21 days) and appears more effective if initiated within the first 3 days of illness.
- Quinolone antibiotics have good in vitro activity against *C. burnetii* and may be used as second line agents.
- Recurrence is treated with a repeat course of doxycycline.

Treatment of chronic Q fever endocarditis

- Chronic Q fever endocarditis is very difficult to treat
- Requires multiple drug combinations: consult microbiologist
- Doxycycline in combination with quinolones for at least 4 years or,
  Doxycycline in combination with hydroxychloroquine for 1.5 to 3 years, which has fewer relapses, but requires routine eye examination to detect accumulation of chloroquine.
- Surgical replacement of damaged cardiac valves may be required for *Coxiella burnetii* endocarditis.

LINKS TO BOOK ONE

1. Case 12, page 35. Mitral stenosis (Prevention of endocarditis).

Case 61

Reversed Arm Leads on ECG

This is the ECG of a 32-year-old man with chest pain.

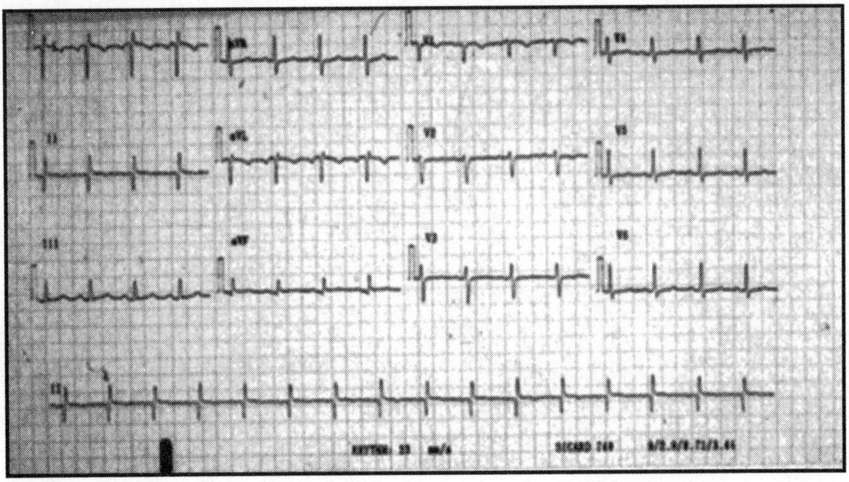

What is the ECG diagnosis?

A. Right ventricular hypertrophy
B. Dextrocardia
C. Reversed arm leads
D. Right bundle branch block
E. Wolff-Parkinson-White syndrome

Answer (C)

DISCUSSION

The main ECG findings are:

- Right axis deviation
- Inverted P and T waves in leads I and aVL
- Tall R wave in lead aVR, but with positive P and T waves

The possible explanations are:

- Dextrocardia
- Reversed arm leads

In dextrocardia the precordial leads show dominant R waves in the right precordial leads and the R waves regress towards the leads V5 and V6. In this patient, the precordial leads show the normal pattern of R wave voltages i.e. progression of the R wave amplitudes towards V5 and V6. Consequently, the correct explanation for the tall R wave in lead aVR in this ECG is reversal of the arm leads.

Case 62

Dilated Cardiomyopathies

This is the transthoracic echocardiogram of a 56-year-old man who presented with breathlessness.

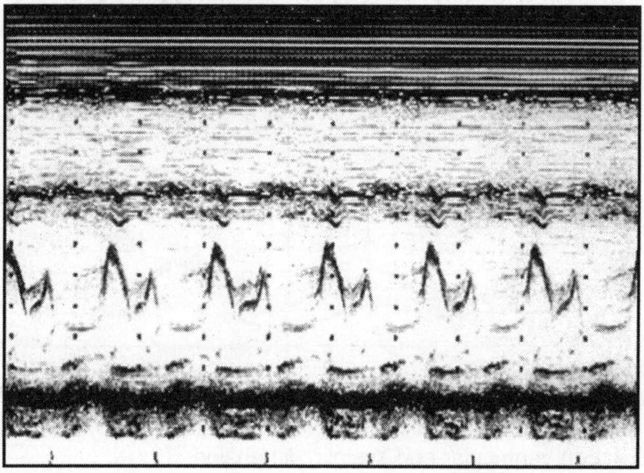

What is the diagnosis?

A. Mitral stenosis
B. Left ventricular hypertrophy
C. Left ventricular dilatation and poor left ventricular function
D. Left ventricular dilatation
E. Right sided cardiomyopathy

Answer (C)

DISCUSSION

This patient's echocardiogram showed a dilated left ventricle with poor left ventricular function. For comparison, a normally functioning left ventricle is shown in Figure 62.1. The shape of the mitral valve is normal and excludes the diagnosis of mitral stenosis.

The absence of fluid accumulation in front of the right ventricle or behind the posterior wall of the left ventricle refutes the diagnosis of pericardial effusion.

An increased awareness of the common echocardiographic abnormalities is gaining importance for acute physicians. Hand held echocardiograph machines are commonly used in emergency rooms and intensive therapy units (ITU). A large pericardial effusion behind the posterior wall of the left ventricle is shown in Figures 62.2 and 62.3.

Dilated Cardiomyopathy

This condition is characterized by left ventricular dilatation and poor

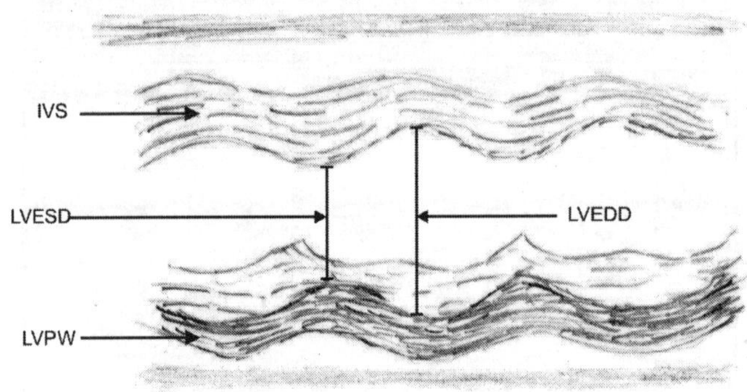

Figure 62.1: Schematic illustration of a normal M-mode echocardiogram
IVS – Interventricular septum
LVESD – Left ventricular end systolic dimension
LVEDD – Left ventricular end diastolic dimension
LVPW – Left ventricular posterior wall

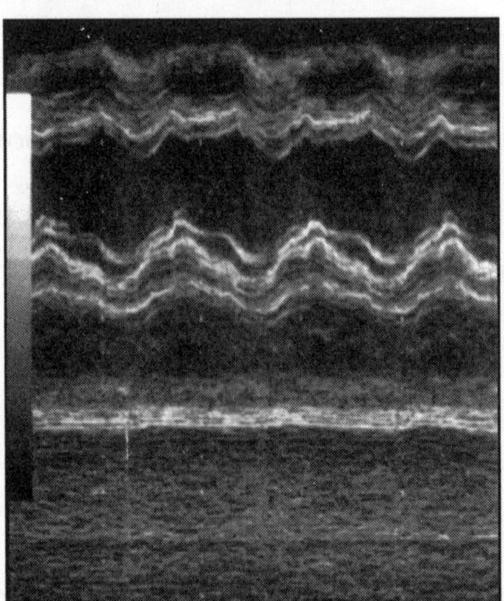

Figure 62.2: Left parasternal view of M-mode echo showing a large pericardial effusion

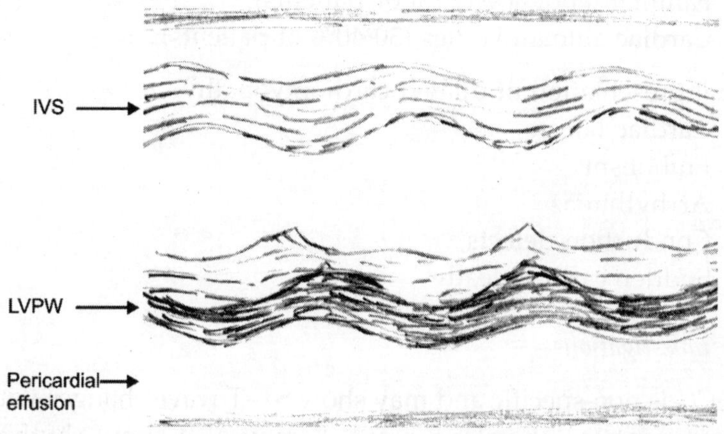

Figure 62.3: Schematic representation of the M-mode echo in Figure 62.2 with the cardiac chamber anatomy and large pericardial effusion highlighted

left ventricular function. The right ventricle may be involved later on in the disease process. Echocardiography is essential for accurate diagnosis.

Secondary causes of dilated cardiomyopathy

- Cardiovascular disease:
  - Ischaemic heart disease
  - Hypertension
  - Rheumatic heart disease
- Alcohol abuse
- Connective tissue diseases such lupus erythematosus, systemic sclerosis
- Amyloidosis
- Cytotoxic drugs, especially doxorubicin and cyclophosphamide
- Muscular dystrophies
- Friedreich's ataxia
- Fabry's disease

Idiopathic dilated cardiomyopathy

The exact cause is not known, but there is a link with the following factors:

- HLA DR-4
- Previous viral infections: Coxsackie virus, HIV

- Familial tendency (20% of patients)
- Cardiac autoantibodies (30-40% of patients).

Clinical presentation of dilated cardiomyopathy

- Cardiac failure
- Embolism
- Arrhythmias
- Conduction defects
- Sudden cardiac death

Other investigations

The ECG is non-specific and may show ST–T wave changes with or without ventricular enlargement. It may also show rhythm or conduction abnormalities. The chest X ray may reveal cardiac enlargement with or without pulmonary congestion.
Treatment of idiopathic dilated cardiomyopathy
Medical treatment includes:

- Anti-failure therapy
- Anticoagulation if there is atrial fibrillation or a history of embolism.
- Avoid alcohol
- Metoprolol has been shown to improve LV function
- Implantable cardiac defibrillator (ICD).
- Cardiac transplantation for suitable patients.

Echocardiographic Left Ventricular Dimensions and Function

Left ventricular function can be measured in terms of:

- Regional wall motion abnormalities (RWMA)
- Ejection fraction estimation

Echocardiogram Reference Values

Left Ventricle	End-systolic		2.5 – 3.8 cm
Wall Thickness	End-diastolic		3.8 - 5.6 cm
	Diastolic	Septum	0.7 - 1.2 cm
		Posterior wall	0.6 - 1.0 cm
	Systolic	Septum	0.9 - 1.8 cm
		Posterior wall	0.9 - 1.8 cm
Fractional Shortening	28 - 44%		
Ejection Fraction	64 - 83 %		
Left Atrium Diameter	2 - 4 cm		

The RWMA are measured by 2-D echocardiogram and important in post myocardial infarct patients. The segments affected by the occluded artery are studied and scored according to the American Society of Cardiology guidelines. These scores give an estimate of the prognosis.

The left ventricular thickness and amplitude of wall motion are studied in the M-mode echocardiogram. From these an estimate of the ejection fraction is calculated. In the absence of RWMA the ejection fraction gives a global estimate of cardiac function.

Case 63

Infections in IV Drug Abusers

A 28-year-old drug addict presented to the A and E department with a one-week history of fever, cough, haemoptysis and excessive tiredness. On examination, the temperature was 39° Celsius, the pulse was irregular with an apex rate of 110 bpm and blood pressure 110/60 mm Hg. There were signs of finger clubbing, raised JVP, right ventricular heave, a pansystolic murmur at the left sternal edge and fine crackles in right lower zone of the chest.

Hb	9.2 g/dl
WBC	18 x 10^9/l
Neutrophil	85%
Na	138 mmol/l
K	5.2 mmol/l
Urea	11.0 mmol/l
Platelets	152 x 10^9/l
Creatinine	113 μmol/l
CRP	350 mg/l
Glucose	7.5 mmol/l
Urinalysis	protein + and blood +
ECG	Atrial fibrillation with RV strain pattern
CXR	Consolidation of the right lower zone with cavitation; and three other small cavities surrounded by patchy consolidation in the left lung.
Blood cultures	Initial verbal report: Gram-positive cocci

What is the next most important investigation?

A. Transthoracic echocardiography
B. Auto-antibody screening

C. Ventilation-perfusion lung scan
D. Sputum culture for AFB
E. Gallium isotope bone scan

Answer (A)

DISCUSSION

Skin and soft tissue infections associated with IV drug abuse

- Cellulitis
- Skin abscess
- Necrotizing fasciitis ± myositis

Skin infections are more common than chest infections or endocarditis. The usual microorganisms are *Staphylococcus aureus* and β-haemolytic streptococci. Other organisms may be involved, including gram-negative bacilli *(Klebsiella, Pseudomonas, Escherichia coli and Proteus)*. Infection of deeper skin layers may lead to abscess formation. Synergy between streptococcal infection and cocaine-induced tissue ischaemia can produce large necrotic ulceration and extensive tissue loss. Necrotizing fasciitis without or with myositis is a dangerous complication.

Pulmonary infections associated with IV drug abuse

- Pneumonia
- Septic pulmonary emboli
- *Mycobacterium tuberculosis*
- Lung abscess or empyema
- Necrotizing pneumonitis
- Pneumocystis carinii pneumonia
- Mediastinitis

Most pulmonary infections are community acquired and due to common respiratory pathogens, such as *Streptococcus pneumoniae*, oral anaerobes, *Staphylococcus aureus* and *Pseudomonas aeruginosa*. Lung abscesses may arise from septic emboli, aspiration pneumonia or necrotizing pneumonitis. Pulmonary tuberculosis is a major problem even in non-HIV-1-infected drug abusers. In addition to infective complications, the lungs in IV drug abusers could be damaged by:

- Starch causing mild transient pulmonary granuloma formation.

- Cotton fibres from drug filters and talc may cause permanent intravascular and perivascular granulomas in pulmonary arteries and arterioles.
- Heroin overdose may be associated with unilateral or bilateral pulmonary oedema.

Bone and joint infections associated with IV drug abuse

- Arthritis
- Osteomyelitis
- Cervical abscess

Any bone or joint can be involved by haematogenous spread. Joint infections usually involve the knees (and the right knee is affected more often than the left). Unusual sites for infective arthritis are the sternoclavicular and costochondral joints and the pubic symphysis. The lumbosacral spine is the most common site of infection in vertebral osteomyelitis. The latter could be complicated by subdural or epidural abscess. Primary sternal osteomyelitis may occur in IV drug abusers.

Cardiovascular infections associated with IV drug abuse

- Endocarditis
- Peripheral vascular infections
- Septic thrombophlebitis
- Mycotic aneurysm
- Arteriovenous fistula
- Thrombosis of internal jugular vein

The most common organisms are Staphylococci (including coagulase-negative strains) and Streptococci (Groups A, B and G). Polymicrobial endocarditis with up to eight pathogens has been described in IV drug abusers. Unusual bacteria in the endocarditis of IV drug users include *Corynebacterium xerosis, Neisseria subflava* and *Neisseria flavescens*. The clinical features of infective endocarditis in IV-drug abuse are different from non-IV-drug abuse. In IV drug abuse patients:

- Valves on the right side (especially the tricuspid valve) of the heart are affected more than the left.
- Septic pulmonary embolism with lung abscesses and cavitations are described.

Central nervous system and eye infection associated with IV drug abuse

- Meningitis
- Encephalitis
- Brain abscess
- Spinal abscess
- Endophthalmitis

Infections of the central nervous system may occur locally or secondary to infection elsewhere such as infective endocarditis. The latter may be complicated by brain abscess, meningitis, and haemorrhage from ruptured mycotic aneurysm. The causative organisms for brain abscess are usually pyogenic bacteria, but other responsible organisms include *Nocardia* and fungi including *Aspergillus* sp, Chaetomium strumarium and mucormycosis.

Splenic abscess associated with IV drug abuse

Splenic abscess could be single or multiple. The causative organisms are commonly Staphylococci, Streptococci, gram-negative bacilli and anaerobes.

Serious viral infections associated with IV drug abuse

- Hepatitis (A, B, C, D, G)
- HIV

Viral hepatitis, including hepatitis A, can be transmitted intravenously. IV drug abuse accounts for about one-quarter of the reported adult cases of AIDS in the United States.

Case 64

Ventricular Fibrillation and CPR

A 66-year-old man was admitted to the CCU with an acute anterior myocardial infarction. He received IV fluids, thrombolysis with tPA, followed by IV heparin for 24 hours and his condition stabilised. On his second day in hospital and while eating his dinner, he suddenly collapsed and the ECG monitor revealed the following tracing.

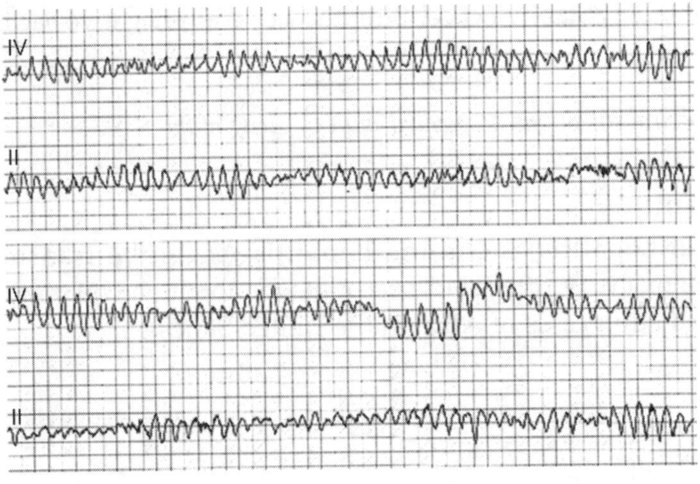

What is the most appropriate immediate management?

A. DC cardioversion
B. Electrical defibrillation
C. IV lignocaine
D. Intravenous bretylium
E. IV amiodarone

Answer (B)

DISCUSSION

Ventricular Fibrillation

The ECG shows ventricular fibrillation, which appears as very rapid and shapeless irregular ventricular activations (or oscillations). These oscillations are sometimes so fine that the ECG tracing may look like a straight line as in asystole.

Cardiac Arrest

Cardiac arrest is the abrupt loss of heart function presenting as loss of consciousness with no signs of breathing or circulation. The underlying rhythm abnormalities are:

- Ventricular fibrillation (VF)
- Pulseless ventricular tachycardia (VT)
- Asystole
- Electromechanical dissociation.

The most common cause of sudden cardiac arrest in adults is ischaemic heart disease. Other causes include primary cardiac arrhythmias and cardiomyopathies. In most patients, the presenting rhythm is ventricular fibrillation or pulseless ventricular tachycardia (Figure 64.1) and electrical defibrillation is the most effective treatment. Ventricular fibrillation may be precipitated by premature ventricular ectopic beats coming on the T wave of the previous cardiac cycle and this is called 'R on T' phenomenon (Figure 64.2).

The non-cardiac conditions that can precipitate a secondary cardiac arrest include:

- Pulmonary embolism
- Tension pneumothorax
- Drug overdose
- Hypovolaemia
- Hypothermia
- Metabolic disturbances (e.g. hypokalaemia, hyperkalaemia)

The above-mentioned conditions are grouped together as electromechanical dissociation wherein there is electrical activity of the heart, but no cardiac output.

The universal ALS algorithm for managing cardiac arrest situations as advised by the resuscitation council (UK) is as follows:

- In cardiac arrest, the airway is cleared and secured. Basic life support (BLS) includes cardiac compression and assisted

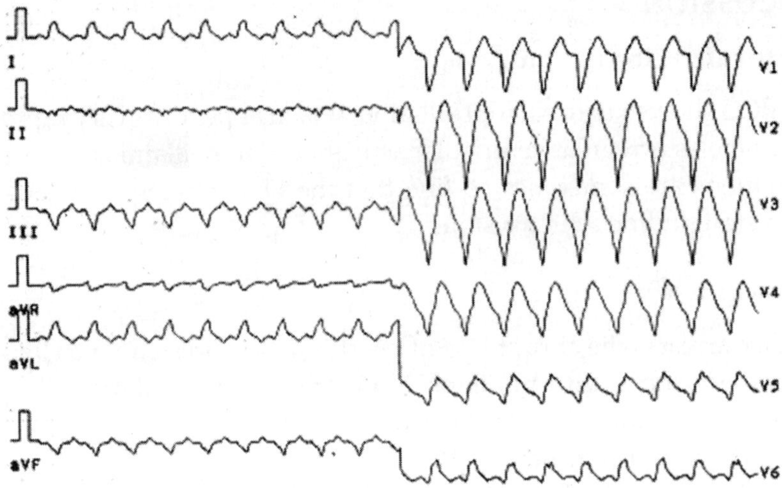

Figure 64.1: Wide complex tachycardia due to ventricular tachycardia

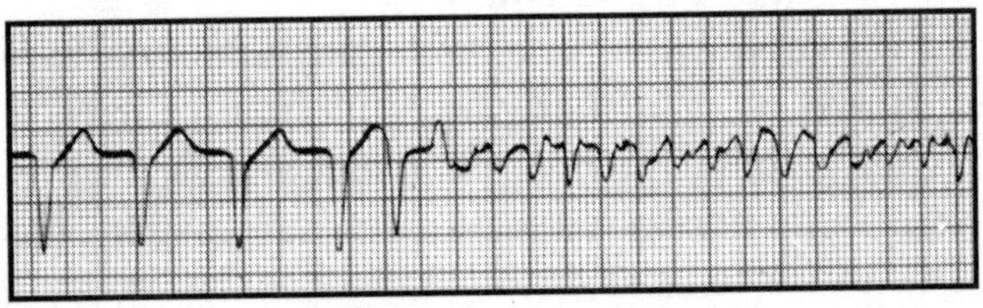

Figure 64.2: 'R on T' phenomena precipitating ventricular fibrillation

ventilation in the ratio of 15:2 establishes breathing and circulation. This is carried on until help arrives for advanced life support (ALS).

LINKS TO BOOK ONE

1. Case 48, page 146. Vasodepressor syncope.
2. Case 53, page 161. Carotid sinus syncope.
3. Case 85, page 287. Torsades-de-pointes tachycardia (Prolonged QT syndromes).

Case 65

Trifascicular Block: Indications for Pacing

A 72-year-old woman with colonic cancer was admitted for an elective left hemicolectomy. The patient has no significant past medical history. The consultant anaesthetist reviewed the preoperative ECG (see below) and diagnosed trifascicular block. He was concerned about complete heart block during the general anaesthetic and asked for a medical review.

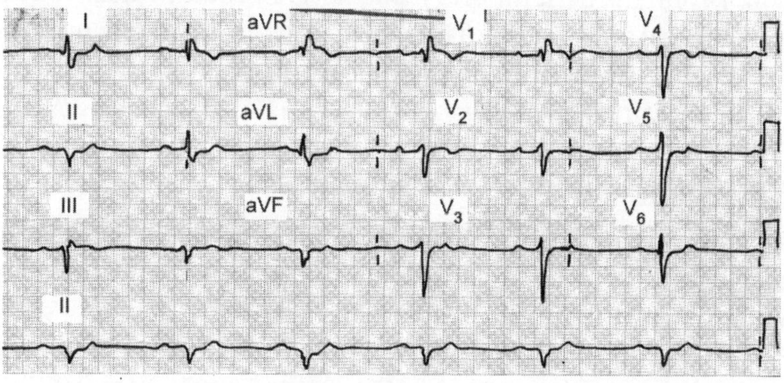

What is the best therapeutic option?

A. Atropine 0.5 mg intravenously as requested
B. Prophylactic temporary pacemaker
C. Prophylactic isoprenaline infusion
D. Postpone the operation until the patient is fitted with a permanent pacemaker
E. Proceed with surgery without any cardiac intervention

Answer (B)

DISCUSSION

This patient has trifascicular block without symptoms. The ECG showed:

- Prolonged PR interval
- Left axis deviation
- Right bundle branch block

Any one of the following also indicates Trifascicular block disease

- Right bundle branch block with alternating left anterior hemiblock or left posterior hemiblock
- Left bundle branch block with alternating right bundle branch block
- Left bundle branch block plus prolonged PR interval

Bifascicular block is diagnosed when:

- Right bundle branch block and left anterior hemiblock, or
- Right bundle branch block and left posterior hemiblock

The incidence of complete heart block (3rd degree AV block) is common in the peri-operative period of patients with trifascicular block, or symptomatic patients with bifascicular block. For this reason, prophylactic temporary pacing is needed in these patients during general anaesthesia. The same applies for patients who have:

- Previous transient complete heart block
- Unexplained syncope

ACC and AHA definitions of evidence for pacing

The American College of Cardiology (ACC) and the American Heart Association (AHA) have defined the types of evidence for pacing (Circulation 1998; 97:1325-1335) and they are as follows:

Class I: Conditions for which there is evidence and/or general agreement that a given procedure or treatment is beneficial, useful, and effective.

Class II: Conditions for which there is conflicting evidence and/or a divergence of opinion about the usefulness/efficacy of a procedure or treatment.

Class IIa: Weight of evidence/opinion is in favour of usefulness/efficacy.

Class IIb: Usefulness/efficacy is less well established by evidence/opinion.

Class III: Conditions for which there is evidence and/or general agreement that a procedure/treatment is not useful/effective and in some cases may be harmful.

Indications for pacing

I *Pacing for Acquired Atrioventricular Block (AV) in Adults*

A. Third-degree AV block at any anatomic level associated with any one of the following conditions:
   - Bradycardia with symptoms presumed to be due to AV block.
   - Arrhythmias and other medical conditions that require drugs that result in symptomatic bradycardia.
   - Documented periods of asystole 3.0 seconds or any escape rate < 40 beats per minute in awake, symptom-free patients.
   - After catheter ablation of the AV junction. There are no trials to assess outcome without pacing, and pacing is virtually always planned in this situation unless the operative procedure is AV junction modification.
   - Postoperative AV block that is not expected to resolve.
   - Neuromuscular diseases with AV block such as myotonic muscular dystrophy, Kearns-Sayre syndrome, Erb's dystrophy (limb-girdle), and peroneal muscular atrophy.

B. Second-degree AV block regardless of type or site of block, with associated symptomatic bradycardia.

II. *Pacing indicated for chronic bifascicular and trifascicular block if associated with*

1. Intermittent third-degree AV block, and/or
2. Type II second-degree AV block.

III. *Pacing for Atrioventricular Block Associated With Acute Myocardial Infarction (AMI)*

1. Persistent second-degree AV block in the His-Purkinje system with bilateral bundle branch block or third-degree AV block within or below the His-Purkinje system after AMI.
2. Transient advanced (second- or third-degree) infranodal AV block and associated bundle branch block. If the site of block is uncertain, an electrophysiological study may be necessary.
3. Persistent and symptomatic second- or third-degree AV block.

IV. *Pacing in Sinus Node Dysfunction*

1. Sinus node dysfunction with documented symptomatic bradycardia, including frequent sinus pauses that produce symptoms. In some patients, bradycardia is iatrogenic and will

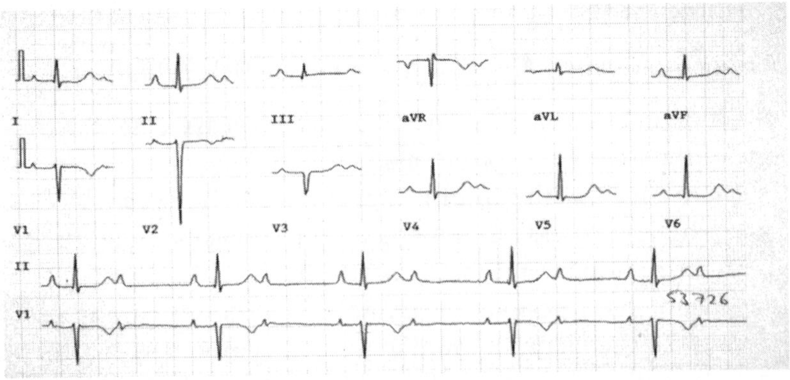

Figure 65.1: Second degree atrioventricular block (Mobitz II)

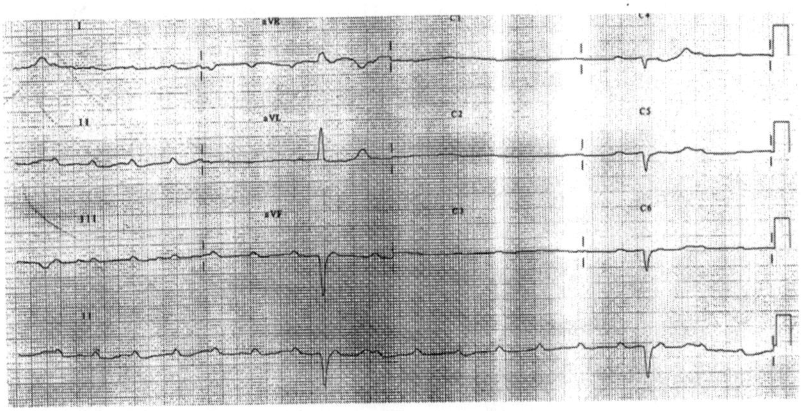

Figure 65.2: Complete (third degree) Atrioventricular (AV) block

occur as a consequence of essential long-term drug therapy of a type and dose for which there are no acceptable alternatives.

2. Symptomatic chronotropic incompetence.

V. *Prevention and Termination of Tachyarrhythmias by Pacing*

1. Symptomatic recurrent supraventricular tachycardia that is reproducibly terminated by pacing after drugs and catheter ablation fail to control the arrhythmia or produce intolerable side effects.
2. Symptomatic recurrent sustained VT as part of an automatic defibrillator system.

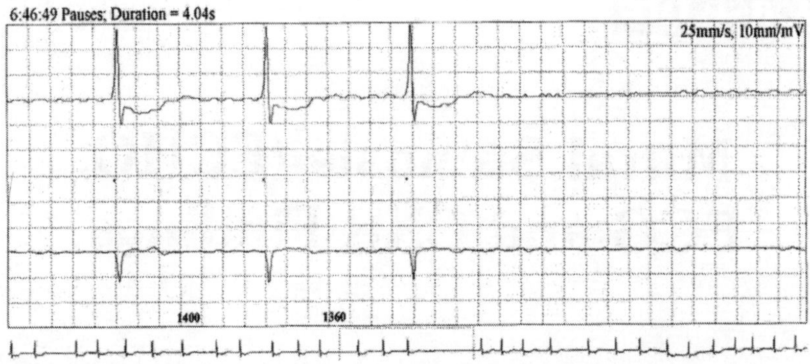

Figure 65.3A: Sick sinus syndrome with a prolonged pause (4.04 seconds)

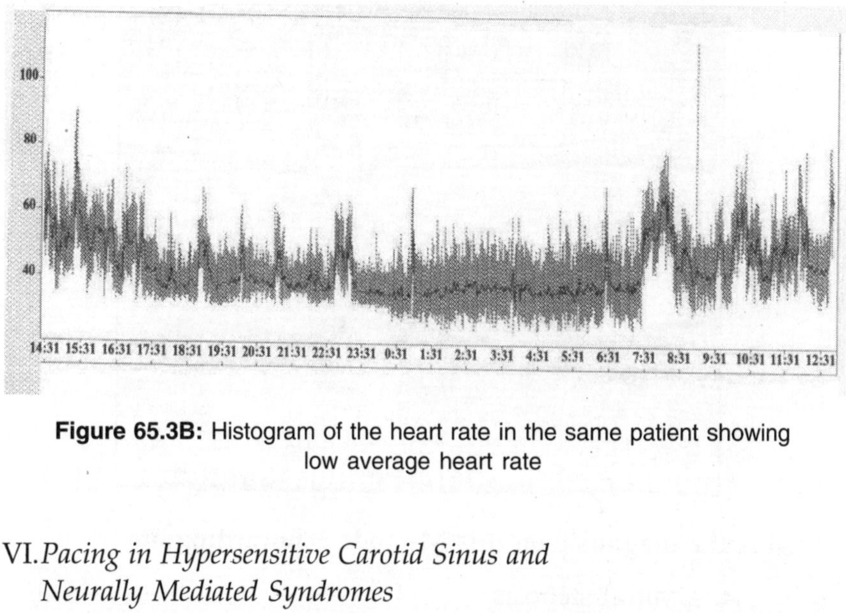

Figure 65.3B: Histogram of the heart rate in the same patient showing low average heart rate

VI. *Pacing in Hypersensitive Carotid Sinus and Neurally Mediated Syndromes*

1. Recurrent syncope caused by carotid sinus stimulation; minimal carotid sinus pressure induces ventricular asystole of >3 Seconds duration in the absence of any medication that depresses the sinus node or AV conduction.

For pacing in Class II indications or specific conditions, please refer to the main article (Circulation 1998; 97:1325-1335). Figures 65.1, 2, and 3 (A and B) show second degree AV block, third degree AV block and a prolonged pause due to sick sinus syndrome respectively. These abnormalities require pacemaker implantation.

Case 66

Mitral Stenosis (ECHO, ECG and CXR Findings)

This is the M-mode echocardiogram of a breathless 56-year-old patient.

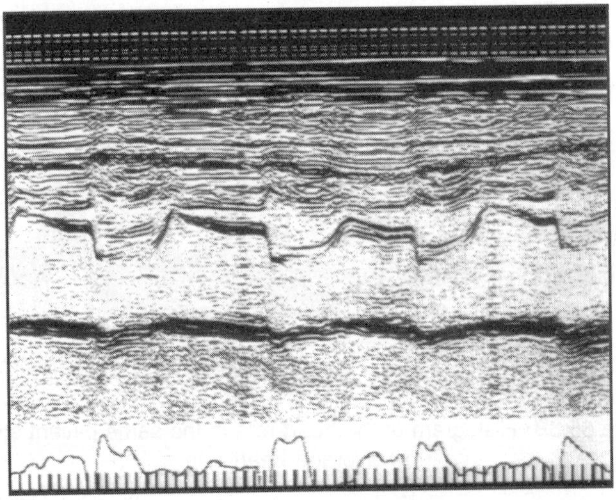

What is the diagnosis on this M-mode echocardiogram?

A. Mitral stenosis
B. Mitral regurgitation
C. Pericardial effusion
D. Aortic stenosis
E. Atrial myxoma

Answer (A)

DISCUSSION

Echocardiographic Features of Mitral Stenosis

Echocardiography uses ultrasound waves to examine the heart. Ultrasound waves have a frequency of > 20 kHz that are not audible to the human ear. They are produced by the piezo-electric effect whereby crystals inter-convert electrical and mechanical oscillations. When ultrasound enters a new medium of different density some of it is reflected back. The returning signals are captured by the crystal and converted back into electrical oscillations, which can be displayed on a monitor or printed out on paper. The different echocardiography methods include 2-D echo, motion (M-mode) echo, or colour Doppler. In motion (M-mode) echo the waves are directed in one plane and are helpful in studying wall chamber thickness and valve mobility. The mitral valve consists of a mitral annulus (ring) to which the two leaflets (anterior and posterior) are attached. The free edges of the leaflets are attached to the chordae tendinae, which are fixed to the left ventricle by papillary muscles. The free edges of the leaflets meet at points called commissures.

During early diastole (E wave), the anterior and posterior leaflets move apart letting blood flow into the ventricles. As the blood flows into the ventricle the leaflets drift towards each other giving rise to the first peak as shown below. The atrial contraction (A wave) sets in next pushing the leaflets apart again resulting in a second peak. Hence, the anterior leaflet produces a 'M' pattern and the posterior leaflet produces a 'W' pattern as shown below.

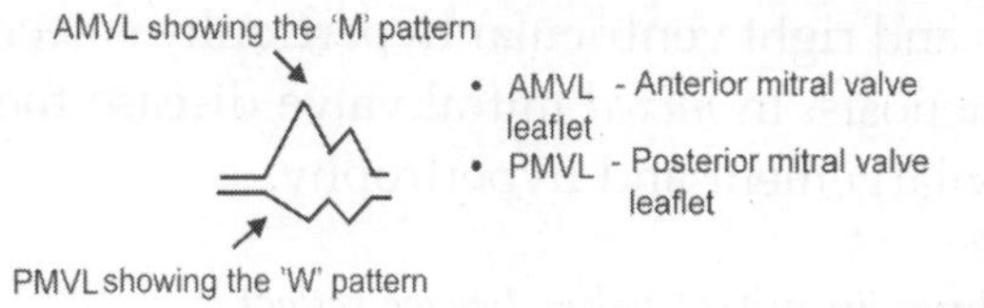

In mitral stenosis, commonly due to rheumatic heart disease, the leaflets are thickened, fibrosed and there is commissural fusion. This prevents the leaflets from moving apart during diastole and results in the loss of the typical echo pattern. In atrial fibrillation the second peak of mitral valve movement is absent. These features are shown below.

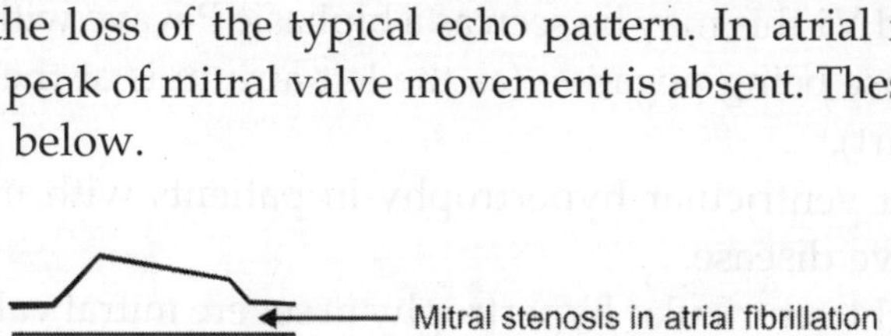

When there is calcification of the mitral valve, the valve leaflets reflect stronger echos compared to the sharp images produced by a normal valve.

Echocardiographic Assessment of Mitral Stenosis

The mitral valve area is normally 4 to 6 cm^2. Mitral stenosis is said to exist when the mitral valve area is < 4 cm^2. The grading of the mitral valve stenosis according to the mitral valve area is as follows:

- Mild 2 - 4 cm^2
- Moderate 1- 2 cm^2
- Severe < 1.0 cm^2

Other criteria for severe mitral stenosis are

- Pressure half time > 200 ms (milliseconds)
- Mean pressure gradient (left atrium to left ventricle) > 10 mmHg
- Systolic pulmonary artery pressure > 35 mmHg

The ECG in Mitral Valve Disease

In *pure* mitral stenosis, there is no left ventricular dilatation or hypertrophy. Left atrial dilatation leading to pulmonary hypertension and right ventricular hypertrophy is seen in advanced *pure* mitral stenosis. In *mixed* mitral valve disease there is also left ventricular enlargement and hypertrophy.

The ECG findings in mitral valve disease reflect

- Rhythm: atrial fibrillation is often present and due to left atrial enlargement or hypertrophy.
- Signs of left atrial enlargement or hypertrophy seen as prolonged bifid P waves particularly in the limb leads, but in lead V1 this may be seen as a biphasic P wave with the second phase being negative (as the left atrium is at the back of the heart).
- Left ventricular hypertrophy in patients with mixed mitral valve disease.
- Right ventricular hypertrophy in severe mitral valve or mixed mitral valve disease (Figure 66.1).

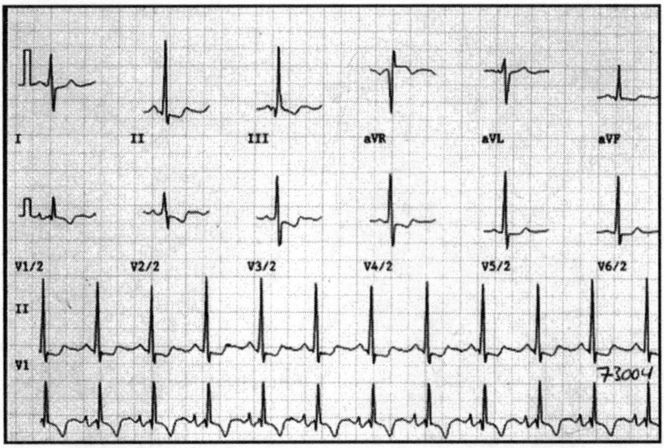

Figure 66.1: Biventricular hypertrophy due to mixed mitral valve disease. The ECG shows sinus rhythm with Sokolow-Lyon precordial voltage criteria of left ventricular hypertrophy (SV1 + RV5 or RV6 ≥ 3.5 mV). There is right axis deviation and the tall R wave with ST-T depression in lead V1 indicates right ventricular hypertrophy.

The Chest X-ray in Mitral Valve Disease

In practice, almost all patients will have a chest X-ray before an echocardiogram. It is important to be familiar with the radiological abnormalities of mitral stenosis and mitral valve disease. Figure 66.2 shows mild enlargement of the pulmonary artery. A prominent main pulmonary artery due to pulmonary hypertension indicates severe mitral valve disease. An earlier change is the prominent left atrial appendage located just below the pulmonary artery. This creates a straight left heart border. In advanced cases (Figure 66.3) and with highly penetrated films, one may see the shadow of the left atrium just inside to the right cardiac border. Other features include:

- Elevation of the left main bronchus (due to enlarged left atrium).
- Mitral valve calcification seen to the left of the spine.
- Dilated upper lobe veins in the erect position (elevated left atrial pressure).
- Prominent vessels in the upper zones (increased pulmonary vascular resistance).
- Kerley B lines in the lower zones (interstitial oedema)
- Basal pleural effusions (pulmonary congestion)
- Interstitial oedema (pulmonary oedema)
- Pulmonary haemosiderosis (chronic pulmonary congestion)
- Enlargement of the right ventricle

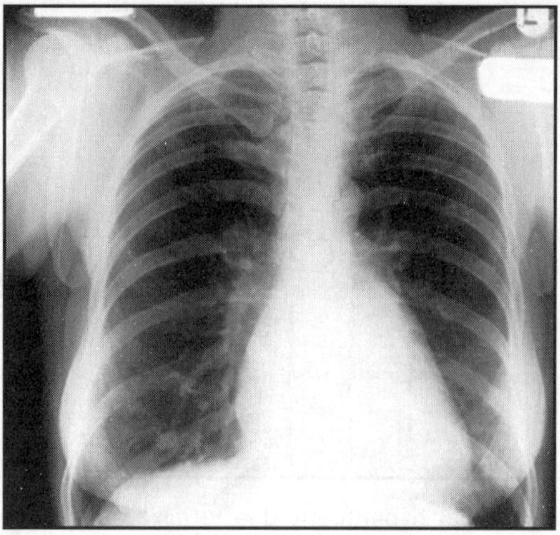

Figure 66.2: Chest X-ray of early mitral valve disease

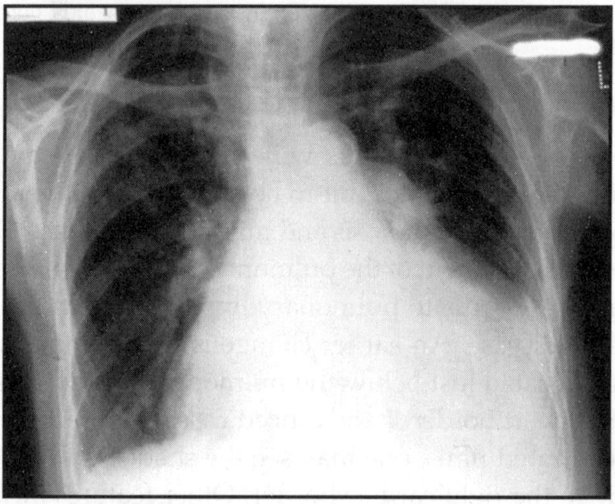

Figure 66.3: Chest X-ray of severe mitral valve disease and cardiac failure

LINKS TO BOOK ONE

1. Case 12, page 35. Mitral stenosis.

Case 67

Cardiac Chamber Masses

Figure 67.1 is the 2-D echocardiogram of a 55-year-old lady who presented with an acutely ischaemic left foot.

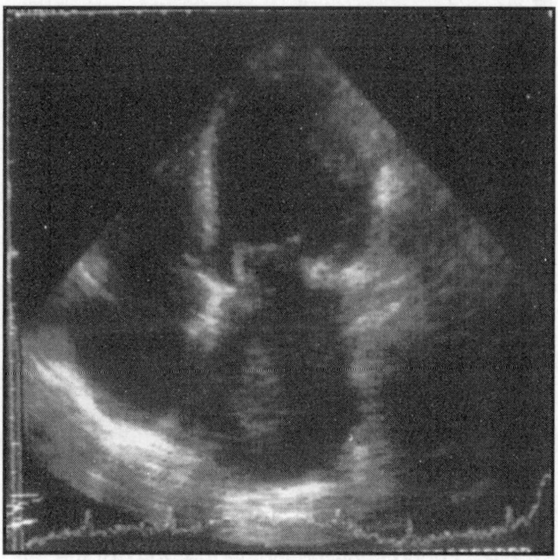

Figure 67.1: 2-D echo

What are the two possible diagnoses?

A. Right ventricular thrombus
B. Atrial septal defect
C. Left atrial myxoma
D. Left atrial thrombus
E. Right atrial thrombus
F. Mitral valve vegetation
G. Right myxoma
H. Left ventricular thrombus

Answer C, D

Intracardiac thrombus

Cavitary thrombus is the most frequent intracardiac mass and commonly occurs in the left atrium or left ventricle. A thrombus occurs when there is stagnation of blood in the cardiac chambers as in atrial fibrillation, in a dilated atrium or ventricle, around prosthetic valves, and after myocardial infarction. Cardiac thrombi are echo bright and usually have clear margins. They need to be distinguished from stagnant blood, cardiac masses, or vegetations in the heart. Figure 67.2 shows the echocardiogram (apical four chamber view) of another patient with a thrombus in the apex of the left ventricle. A schematic illustration of the cardiac anatomy in a four-chamber view is shown in Figures 67.3 and 67.4.

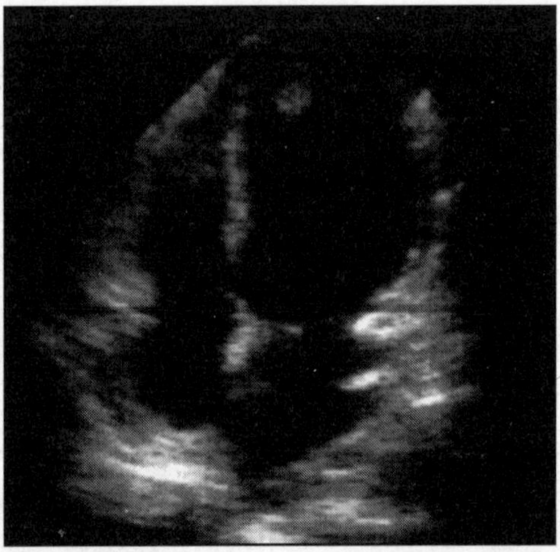

Figure 67.2: 2-D echo showing clot in the apex of the left ventricle

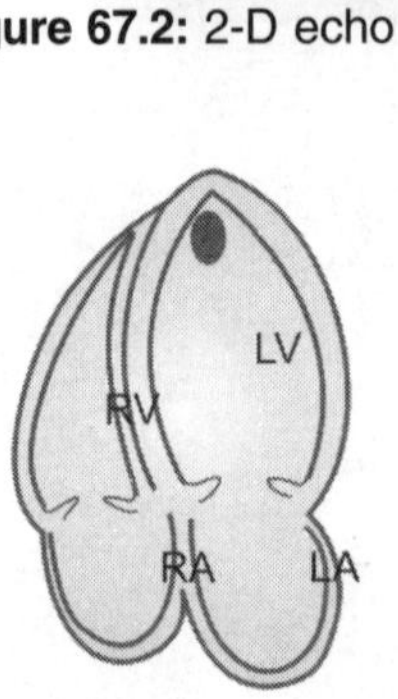

Figure 67.3: A schematic diagram of figure 67.2 and its four-chamber view (2 – D echo) of a left ventricular thrombus

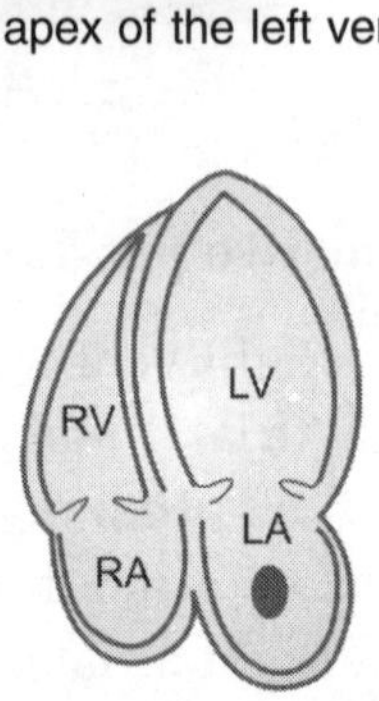

Figure 67.4: A schematic diagram of figure 67.1 and its four-chamber view (2 – D echo) of a left atrial thrombus

Differential Diagnosis of Cardiac Masses

Echocardiography is important in identifying the position, size, mobility and nature of masses in the heart. These include:

- Thrombi
- Vegetations
- Primary tumours
  - Benign (myxoma, lipoma, rhabdomyoma): atrial myxoma is the commonest cardiac tumour.
  - Malignant (sarcoma)
- Secondary tumours originating from the lung, kidney and haematological malignancies are more common than primary cardiac tumours. They may be direct extensions from the lungs or mediastinum, or metastatic. Cardiac tumours in patients with AIDS are usually Kaposi's sarcoma or lymphoma.

Case 68

Acute Myocardial Infarction

This 82-year-old man presented with chest pain of two hours duration. He was given oxygen and intravenous diamorphine. The ECG on admission is shown below.

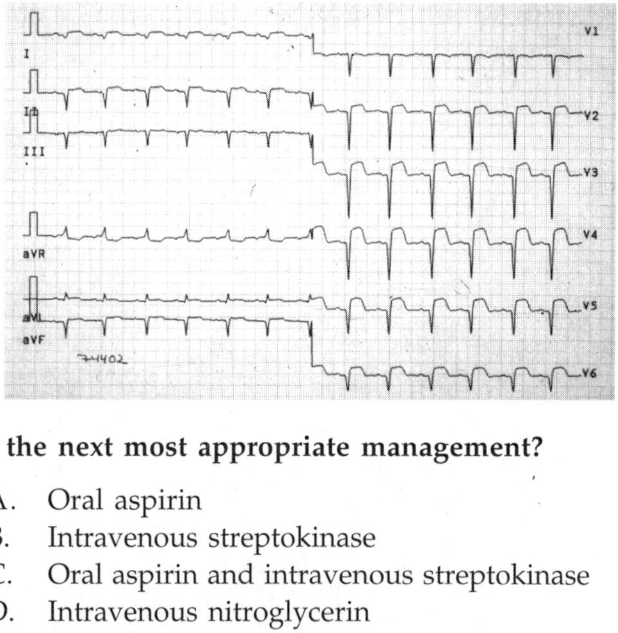

What is the next most appropriate management?

A. Oral aspirin
B. Intravenous streptokinase
C. Oral aspirin and intravenous streptokinase
D. Intravenous nitroglycerin
E. Warfarin

Answer (C)

DISCUSSION

The Management of Acute Myocardial Infarction

The ECG showed ST-segment elevation consistent with acute anteroseptal myocardial infarction. For comparison Figure 68.1 shows the changes in an acute inferior myocardial infarction. The management of acute myocardial infarction includes pain relief with intravenous diamorphine (with or without anti-emetic drugs), oxygen, bed rest, monitoring in a coronary care unit, and treatment of any complications. The ultimate aim is to reduce mortality by the combined use of aspirin (loading dose of 300 mg) and thrombolysis. Although this patient is elderly, old age per se is not a barrier to active treatment and many centres would be happy to give streptokinase infusion (1.5 mega units over about one hour). This regime will not require heparin subsequently.

Other important measures are:

- Continue aspirin orally (75-150 mg od)
- Statins (check serum cholesterol on admission)
- If not contraindicated, beta-blockers and ACE inhibitor (e.g. ramipril)

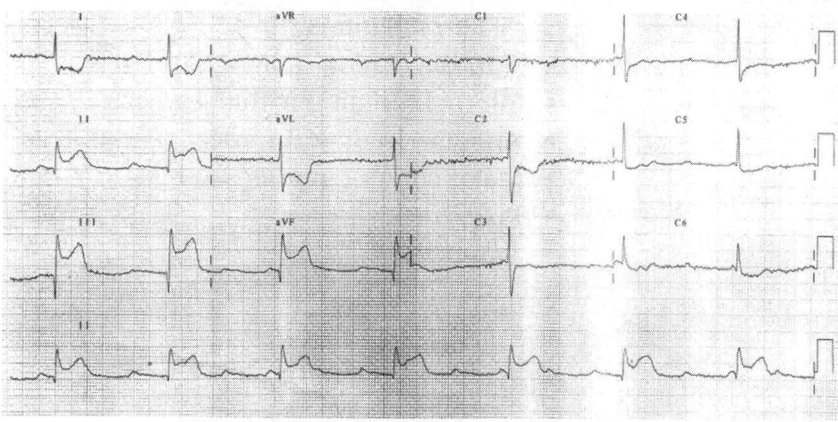

Figure 68.1: Acute inferior myocardial infarction

This ECG shows ST segment elevation in leads II, III and AVF, which is typical of acute inferior myocardial infarction due to occlusion of the right coronary artery. There is also ST depression in leads I, AVL and V2 – such changes are often referred to as "reciprocal" and could indicate concomitant stenotic disease in the left coronary artery.

Indications for Thrombolysis in Acute Myocardial Infarction

1. Chest pain suggestive of myocardial infarction and presentation within 12 hours and:
   - ST elevation ≥ 0.2 mV in 2 adjacent chest leads

     or

- ST elevation $\geq$ 0.1 mV in 2 or more limb leads

  or
- Dominant R and ST depression in V1-V3 (posterior infarct)

  or
- New-onset left bundle branch block

2. Presentation 12-24 hours after onset of cardiac chest pain with continuing pain +/- ECG evidence of evolving infarct

Contraindications to Thrombolysis

Absolute	• Prior haemorrhagic stroke • CVA during prior 6 months • Active internal bleeding • Aortic dissection
Relative	• Severe uncontrolled hypertension (> 180/110 mmHg) • Anticoagulation (INR > 2.5) • Internal bleeding within 4 weeks • Known bleeding disorder • Major surgery in prior 4 weeks • Pregnancy • Traumatic CPR

Case 69

Hypertensive Encephalopathy

A 72-year-old man was brought to the A and E by his wife at 10 pm. He had been confused and had two fits in the last 24 hours. Hypertension was diagnosed 5 years ago and has been under control with medication. He was teetotal and did not smoke. In the A and E, his pulse was regular at 78 bpm and blood pressure 240/140 mmHg. Neurologically he was alert without signs of meningeal irritation. The deep tendon reflexes were exaggerated, but the plantar responses were flexor. Fundoscopy showed flame shaped retinal haemorrhages, soft exudates and papilloedema. There was no focal motor deficit. An urgent CT brain was normal.

What is the most likely diagnosis?

A. Subarachnoid haemorrhage
B. Benign intracranial hypertension
C. Communicating hydrocephalus
D. Hypertensive encephalopathy
E. Severe hypertension

Answer (D)

DISCUSSION

Malignant Hypertension

There is some controversy in the definition for accelerated hypertension and malignant hypertension. Accelerated hypertension is 'severe hypertension with bilateral retinal haemorrhages and exudates, but without papilloedema'. The term malignant hypertension is then reserved for 'severe hypertension with papilloedema'. Some authors do not make this distinction, because the pathology (see below) is similar in both conditions and the finding of papilloedema is of no additional prognostic value.

- The diastolic blood pressure in malignant hypertension is generally > 120-130 mmHg, but there is no absolute value above which malignant hypertension always develops and below which it never occurs.
- Malignant hypertension is commoner in blacks, cigarette smokers, renal disease, renovascular disease, IgA nephropathy.
- Fibrinoid necrosis and subintimal cellular proliferation are characteristic features of malignant hypertension. These vascular changes inevitably cause narrowing of the arteriolar lumen and tissue ischaemia.
- Activation of the clotting system leads to fibrin strands being formed within the arteriolar lumen, which cause mechanical damage to red cells or microangiopathic haemolytic anaemia
- Without treatment, the one year mortality is 90 per cent. The causes of death are stroke, renal failure and cardiac failure.

Hypertensive encephalopathy

Hypertensive encephalopathy describes a syndrome of fluctuating neurological symptoms and signs due to malignant hypertension, arterial hyperperfusion, breakdown in the blood brain barrier and cerebral oedema.

- Arterial autoregulation in normotensive people maintains cerebral blood flow constant over a mean arterial pressure of 60-120 mmHg.
- A sudden rapid rise in mean blood pressure above 120 mmHg will overwhelm arterial autoregulation and lead to arteriolar dilatation, increased cerebral blood flow, breakdown in the blood brain barrier and formation of cerebral oedema. This is why hypertensive encephalopathy can occur at lower blood pressures in previously normotensive subjects if there is a large increase in blood pressure over a short time span, as in glomerulonephritis and pre-eclampsia.
- In chronic hypertension, arterial autoregulation is reset upwards so that cerebral blood flow is held constant over a mean arterial pressure of 120-160 mmHg. Consequently,

failure of autoregulation and hypertensive encephalopathy will only occur if mean arterial blood pressures are above 160 mmHg.

Symptoms and signs of hypertensive encephalopathy

- Generalised headache
- Confusion
- Convulsions
- Coma
- Cortical blindness
- Hemiparesis
- Hemisensory loss
- Papilloedema, retinal haemorrhages and exudates

Diagnosis

The key diagnostic features of hypertensive encephalopathy are:

- Fluctuation in neurological signs
- Resolution of symptoms and signs with blood pressure lowering
- Hypertension with papilloedema, retinal haemorrhages and exudates
- Conditions such as pre-eclampsia, eclampsia, phaeochromocytoma, acute glomerulonephritis, renovascular hypertension
- Exclusion of other forms of encephalopathy e.g. diffuse brain injury associated with uraemia, hyponatraemia, drug intoxication (cocaine and amphetamine), encephalitis, vasculitis (as in lupus cerebral vasculitis). Therefore, CT brain scan, blood count (haemolysis), serum chemistry, toxicology, chest X-ray (cardiomegaly) and ECG (LVH) should be requested.

Treatment

Gradually lower the mean arterial blood pressure by 25 per cent over 48 hours. Avoid sudden drops in blood pressure.

- IV nitroprusside (e.g. 0.5-1 μg/kg/min). This has a rapid onset (1 minute) and short duration of action (less than 5 minutes). Cyanide toxicity can occur in uraemic patients and during prolonged IV infusions.

- IV nitrates (e.g. 5 µg/min) can be tried but may produce too rapid a drop in blood pressure
- IV labetolol (e.g. 2mg/min)
- IV hydralazine 5-10 mg over 20 minutes followed by 50-300 mcg/min infusion

LINKS TO BOOK ONE

1. Case 94, page 324. Ambulatory blood pressure profile: non-dipper.
2. Case 97, page 336. White coat hypertension.

Case 70

Ischaemic Stroke

A 67-year-old man whilst driving suddenly lost the use in his left arm, but managed to stop the car. In the car mirror, he also noticed drooping of his left face. The weakness lasted only 10 minutes. His wife convinced him to seek advice. He attended the accident and emergency department two weeks later. There were no current symptoms. He was right handed with no focal limb weakness or cerebellar signs and his gait was normal. His heart rate was 80 bpm (regular rhythm) and the blood pressure was 180/110 mmHg. There were no signs of carotid arterial bruits, valvular heart disease, or heart failure. The CT brain scan was normal.

What is the most appropriate action?

A. Lower the blood pressure urgently with intravenous glyceryl trinitrate
B. Initiate aspirin 300 mg as starting dose followed by 150 mg od
C. Prescribe dipyridamole 100 mg tds
D. Admit the patient for anticoagulation
E. Reassure the patient and arrange follow-up in the neurovascular clinic

Answer (B)

DISCUSSION

This patient has had transient ischaemic attack (TIA). The CT scan of the brain was normal. His heart was in sinus rhythm without clinical evidence of embolisation elsewhere. The main aspects of management are:

1. Urgent referral to a neurovascular clinic within two weeks. However, immediate referral to hospital for urgent assessment is indicated in the following circumstances:
   - Crescendo TIA: the patient has had more than one TIA within a short period
   - Patients are on anticoagulants
   - Complex neurological signs
   - Severe headaches
   - Signs of increased intracranial pressure
2. Cerebral imaging. This is indicated to exclude:
   - Primary intracranial haemorrhage
   - Arterio-venous malformation
   - Subdural haematoma
   - Tumours

   The diagnostic yield of CT brain scan in patients with TIA is small, but a routine policy of non-scanning may miss up to five per cent of serious pathological conditions mentioned above. Urgent scanning is required if patients are on anticoagulation.
3. Modifying the risk factors. All the patients should be assessed for other vascular risk factors and be treated or advised appropriately. This should include advice about life style changes (smoking, diet, exercises, etc). In addition, the following specific risk factors are dealt with:
   a. Hypertension should be managed appropriately. The British Hypertension Society guidelines are: optimal blood pressure treatment targets are systolic blood pressure < 140 mm Hg and diastolic blood pressure < 85 mm Hg; the minimum accepted level of control recommended is < 150 and < 90 mm Hg respectively. For patients with diabetes the target level of control should be 130/80 mm Hg. Further reduction of blood pressure should be considered using a combination of long-acting ACE inhibitor (e.g. perindopril or ramipril) and a thiazide diuretic (e.g. Indapamide).
   b. All patients with TIA's (or ischaemic stroke) who are not on anticoagulation should be taking an antiplatelet agent, i.e. aspirin (75 - 300 mg) daily, or clopidogrel, or a combination of low-dose aspirin and dipyridamole modified release (MR). Where patients are aspirin intolerant an alternative antiplatelet agent (clopidogrel 75 mg daily or dipyridamole MR 200 mg twice daily) should be used.

c. Therapy with a statin should be considered for all patients with a history of ischaemic heart disease and a cholesterol > 5.0 mmol/l following stroke.

d. Anticoagulation. This should not be used after transient ischaemic attacks or minor strokes who are in sinus rhythm unless cardiac embolism is suspected. However, anticoagulation is indicated in every patient who has atrial fibrillation (valvular or non-valvular) unless contraindicated. Primary intra-cranial haemorrhage should be excluded by CT scan of the head prior to anticoagulation.

e. Carotid endarterectomy. Any patient with a hemispheric or ophthalmic TIA or ischaemic stroke (minor or recovered with absent residual disability) should be assessed for carotid endarterectomy. Carotid stenosis $\geq$ 70 per cent measured by Doppler ultrasound on the symptomatic side should be considered for carotid endarterectomy.

LINKS TO BOOK ONE

1. Case 88, page 298. Carotid artery dissection.
2. Case 91, page 309. Stroke in a young patient.

Case 71

Wernicke's Encephalopathy

A 46-year-old unemployed divorcee who lived alone was brought to A and E by his girlfriend. He has been drinking and smoking heavily. In the last few weeks, he has been intermittently confused and unable to sleep at night. On examination, he was disorientated and had a slightly ataxic gait. The SHO started him on an IV five per cent glucose infusion pending review by the medical registrar. Four hours later, the patient's condition had deteriorated. He was now drowsy, but rousable, and there were no eye movements or neck stiffness.

Hb	11.2 g/dl
WBC	$8.0 \times 10^9/l$
Platelets	$192 \times 10^9/l$
Na	129 mmol/l
K	3.2 mmol/l
Urea	4.0 mmol/l
Creatinine	121 µmol/l
Glucose	5.6 mmol/l
Bilirubin	18 µmol/l
Total protein	72 g/dl
Albumin	28 g/dl
ALT	18 U/l
ALP	186 U/l
CXR	normal
ECG	normal

Which are the two most appropriate immediate management measures?

A. Rapid detoxication with diazepam
B. Intravenous cefotaxime to cover for meningitis

C. High dose intravenous thiamine
D. Urgent EEG
E. Psychiatric referral
F. CT scan of the brain
G. MR angiography of the extracranial vessels
H. Temporal lobe biopsy

Answers (C, F)

DISCUSSION

Patients with alcoholism can become unconscious for a variety of reasons, including alcohol intoxication, hypogylcaemia, hepatic failure and Wernicke's encephalopathy. Other conditions unrelated to ethanol abuse needs to be also excluded. Falls are common and may result in brain injury and subdural haematoma. Other primary brain problems that need to be excluded are stroke and tumour.

This patient has a normal blood glucose level and there were no features of hepatic failure. The liver functions tests were reasonable. A CT scan was done and it did not show a focal lesion. The most likely diagnosis is Wernicke's encephalopathy, which was probably precipitated by IV glucose without thiamine supplementation.

Wernicke's Encephalopathy

Wernicke's encephalopathy is an acute neuropsychiatric condition characterized by deficiency of intracellular thiamine (Vitamin B_1) in the brain cells. As a result, there will be cellular energy deficit, focal acidosis, a regional increase in glutamate and ultimately cell death. These brain changes are initially reversible. Pathologically there is necrosis and small haemorrhages predominantly in the periaqueductal midbrain, thalamus, hypothalamus, mammillary bodies, the floor of the fourth ventricle and the cerebellar cortex.

The most common cause of Wernicke's encephalopathy is alcohol abuse (90% of the cases). *The onset is sudden often presenting like a brain stem stroke.* The cardinal signs are:

- Ocular palsies
- Paralysis of abduction of eyes, or paralysis of conjugate lateral gaze
- Nystagmus
- Ataxia

- Mental confusion
- Retinal haemorrhages (papilloedema is unusual)

The classical triad of confusion, ocular palsy (abducens and conjugate) with nystagmus, and ataxia of gait is not common and is only observed in ten percent of patients.

Wernicke's encephalopathy is under diagnosed. It is found in 1.5 per cent of postmortems in general hospitals, but the prevalence from postmortem in alcoholic patients increases to 12.5 per cent and to 30 per cent if thiamine related cerebellar damage is included. Failure to diagnose Wernicke's encephalopathy and institute adequate parenteral therapy will result in death in 20 per cent of patients. Seventy five per cent will be left with permanent brain damage involving short-term memory loss - Korsakoff's psychosis. Twenty five per cent will require long-term institutionalization. The most important measure is prevention. Alcoholic patients have serious thiamine and other vitamin deficiencies because of:

- Inadequate intake
- Loss of thiamine through vomiting or diarrhoea
- Reduced thiamine storage due to liver damage
- Ethanol and malnutrition cause significant inhibition of the active transport mechanism involved in the intestinal absorption of thiamine.

Oral thiamine treatment is not adequate. At risk patients should be giving intravenous multivitamin preparation and thiamine such as Pabrinex. In summary, avoid giving IV glucose without vitamins in at risk patients as it may precipitate Wernicke's encephalopathy.

Case 72

Malaria Prophylaxis in Pregnancy

A 30-year-old housewife from the Middle East was planning to visit her family next year during the spring and summer season. She knew that malaria was prevalent in that area. She was also planning to become pregnant in January or February of the same year. As she has not seen her parents for the past ten years, she planned to stay with them for about 3 to 4 months.

What is the safest malarial prophylaxis assuming that there are no resistant strains?

A. Chloroquine 300 mg weekly and proguanil 200 mg daily
B. Maloprims (dapsone + pyrimethamine)
C. Doxycycline
D. Mefloquine
E. Dapsone alone

Answer (A)

DISCUSSION

Prevention of malaria in pregnancy

- Chloroquine 300 mg weekly is safe.
- Proguanil 200 mg daily is safe, but pregnant women will need folic acid supplement.
- Mefloquine is teratogenic in mice and its safety in pregnancy is not established. It is also excreted in breast milk.
- Doxycycline like all tetracyclines is contraindicated in pregnancy.
- Dapsone-pyrimethamine combination is not safe in pregnancy. It is safe during lactation. It causes folate deficiency

and hence, folate supplement is needed.

Treatment of malaria in pregnancy

- Chloroquine is safe. Both chloroquine and proguanil may be used to prevent relapses.
- Quinine (oral or IV) is also safe in pregnancy. However, parenteral quinine may cause hypoglycaemia.
- Mefloquine is probably safe after the first trimester for the foetus, but it may cause neurological side-effects in mothers.
- Both maloprim and primaquine are unsafe.

Travel vaccinations in pregnancy

Live vaccines stimulate the immune system and provide protection against a specific infection without causing clinical infection, although subclinical infection may occur. *Live vaccine should be avoided in pregnancy, as there is danger of foetal infection.*

Live vaccines

- Bacillus Calmette-Guérin (BCG)
- Measles
- Mumps
- Oral polio vaccine (Sabin)
- Rubella
- Oral typhoid vaccine (TY 21a)
- Yellow fever vaccine

Inactivated vaccines, extracts or toxoids

The inactivated killed organisms are thought to pose little risk to the foetus, but the absolute risk is not zero. Therefore, inactivated killed vaccines should be avoided during pregnancy and used only if they are absolutely necessary.

- Anthrax
- Botulinum toxin
- Cholera
- Pertussus
- Typhoid (whole cell and Vi antigen)
- Meningococci (A and C)
- Pneumococcal pneumonia vaccine
- Hepatitis A (inactivated but not safe in pregnancy - use

immunoglobulin)
- Hepatitis B (Recombinant vaccine)
- Influenza vaccine
- Poliomyelitis (Salk)
- Rabies vaccine
- Diphtheria toxoid
- Tetanus toxoid
- All immunoglobulins

Regime for malaria prophylaxis

Chloroquine 300 mg per week and / or proguanil 200 mg per day for two weeks before and for four weeks after leaving the endemic area. Seek specialist advice in cases from parts of the world where there is chloroquine resistance.

Specific instructions on some vaccinations during pregnancy

* Rubella	Avoid
* Measles	Avoid
* Oral Poliomyelitis (Sabin)	Avoid
* High risk of poliomyelitis	Pregnant women without adequate immunity who are travelling to endemic areas are advised to take the inactivated parenteral (Salk) vaccine.
* Hepatitis A	There is insufficient evidence for the safety of the Hepatitis A vaccine during pregnancy. Therefore, it should be avoided. Instead, use human immunoglobulins.
* Hepatitis B	Pregnant women at risk should take this vaccine.
* Yellow fever	This vaccine is associated with a small risk of encephalitis when given to children < 9 months of age. The same risk is possible in the foetus. Pregnant women travelling to West or Central Africa are at high risk of yellow fever and should carefully evaluate the risks and benefits of vaccination.
* Cholera	No specific contraindication in pregnancy. Cholera vaccination is only effective in 50 per cent of people. General hygiene for water and food may be effective.
* Meningitis	It is advisable to take the vaccine if travelling to an area where there is an epidemic of meningococcal meningitis A or C.
* Typhoid	Live vaccines are contraindicated. If the risk of infection is high, such as travellers to the Indian sub-continent, a single dose of the Vi polysaccharide vaccine is advised.

Case 73

Hypertension in Pregnancy

A 38-year-old primigravida who was 12 weeks pregnant was found to be hypertensive at the antenatal clinic. There was no previous hypertension, renal disease or endocrine disorder. The blood pressure was 160/104 mm Hg and urinalysis was unremarkable.

Which of the following medications would be the safest treatment for her hypertension?

A. Bendroflumethiazide
B. Enalapril
C. Candesartan
D. Nifedipine
E. Minoxidil

Answer (D)

DISCUSSION

ACE-I's and ARB's are contraindicated in pregnancy. Bendroflumethiazide can cause foetal thrombocytopenia. Nifedipine in the dose of 10 mg tds is safe in pregnancy. Other 'safe' antihypertensive drugs in pregnancy are:

- Methyldopa 250 mg bd or tds
- Labetolol 100-400 mg bd

Note: Beta-blockers (e.g. atenolol) may be associated with intra-uterine growth retardation.

Causes of hypertension during pregnancy

BP > 140/90 mmHg before 20 weeks of gestation	a. Known chronic hypertension due to: – Essential hypertension – Renal hypertension – Renovascular hypertension (fibromuscular hyperplasia) – Phaeochromocytoma b. Presumed chronic hypertension
BP > 140/90 mmHg after 20 weeks of gestation	a. Chronic hypertension b. Mild non proteinuria pre-eclampsia c. Proteinuric pre-eclampsia d. Pre-eclampsia complicating chronic hypertension

Pre-existing hypertension in pregnancy

- Pre-existing hypertensive women are 3 times more liable to develop pre-eclampsia during pregnancy (the pre-eclampsia rate is 50%)
- Chronic hypertension also causes intra-uterine growth retardation
- Treatment of chronic hypertension does not prevent pre-eclampsia or foetal growth retardation, but it is indicated for the welfare of the mother.

Pre-eclampsia

- Pre-eclampsia typically occurs after 20 weeks of pregnancy, but may occur earlier in multiple pregnancy and hydatidiform mole.
- Pre-eclampsia is cured by delivery of the baby
- The recurrence of pre-eclampsia or eclampsia is 20 per cent in a subsequent pregnancy.

Diagnosis of pre-eclampsia

The diagnosis is based upon one of the following after 20 weeks of gestation in a woman with previously normal blood pressure:

- Systolic blood pressure ≥140 mm Hg
- Diastolic blood pressure ≥ 90 mm Hg and
- Proteinuria of ≥ 300 mg in a 24-hour urine collection

Symptoms of pre-eclampsia

- Generally no symptoms
- The symptoms include headaches, visual symptoms (flashing lights), vomiting, epigastric pain and oedema.

Predisposing factors for pre-eclampsia

- Primigravida and multipara > 3
- Teenage mothers and older mothers
- Twin pregnancy
- Hydatidiform mole
- Previous hypertension
- Diabetes mellitus
- Previous oral contraceptive pill use
- Low social class

Complications of pre-eclampsia

Maternal complications	• Renal failure • Stroke • Eclamptic fits • Hyper-reflexia • Hepatic failure • Retinal detachment • Papilloedema: retinal haemorrhages and HELLP syndrome: haemolysis, elevated liver enzymes and low platelets.
Foetal complications	• Placental insufficiency and infarction • Intra-uterine growth retardation • Intra-uterine death • Necessity for early delivery: neonatal pulmonary insufficiency can be reduced by giving the mother dexamethasone (an IM 12 mg dose which is repeated once 12 hours later)

Management of pre-eclampsia

- Admission to hospital for bed rest and monitoring
- Blood pressure control: methyldopa, nifedipine or labetolol (see above)
- Expedite delivery of baby
- Avoid ergometrine in the third stage as it can increase blood pressure

Eclampsia

- Diazepam for the initial control of convulsive seizures
- Magnesium sulphate is the drug of choice for preventing further convulsions (typically 4 g over 10 minutes IV followed by an IV infusion of 1 g per hour). Measure plasma magnesium levels (therapeutic range is 2-5 mg/100ml)
- Reduce blood pressure: IV hydralazine 5mg over 15 minutes (may be repeated to a maximum of 20 mg) or labetolol infusion
- Fluid balance
- Expedite delivery of the baby.

LINKS TO BOOK ONE

1. Case 94, page 324. Ambulatory blood pressure profile: non-dipper.
2. Case 97, page 336. White coat hypertension.

Case 74

Indomethacin and Heart Failure

A 68-year-old retired engineer developed acute lumbago and attended the casualty, where an X-ray showed degenerative changes in the lumbar region. His past medical history included: myocardial infarction two years ago, hypercholesterolaemia 10 years ago and hypertension 12 years ago. Heart failure was diagnosed two years after his MI and after treatment, he was walking one mile a day. He was an ex-smoker and drank one glass of wine per day. His current medications included aspirin 75 mg od, pravastatin 40 mg od, isosorbide mononitrate 20 mg bd, atenolol 50 mg od, ramipril 10 mg od and furosemide 40 mg od.

His backache settled within two days with indomethacin 25 mg tds and bed rest. Two weeks later, he awoke from sleep with breathlessness and attended A and E. There was no chest pain. The heart rate was regular at 110 bpm and blood pressure 110/70 mmHg. There was a third heart sound, crackles in the base of both lungs, and pitting ankle oedema. The chest X-ray showed cardiomegaly, pulmonary oedema, and a small right pleural effusion. The ECG showed left bundle branch block.

Na	134 mmol/l
K	5.2 mmol/l
Urea	10.2 mmol/l
Creatinine	140 μmol/l
Glucose	6.2 mmol/l
CRP	< 8 mg/l
CK	150 U/l
Troponin T	< 0.01 μg/l

What is the most likely cause of his cardiac decompensation?

A. Acute MI
B. Chest infection
C. Pulmonary embolism
D. Acute pericarditis
E. Fluid retention due to indomethacin

Answer (E)

DISCUSSION

Any of the conditions listed above can cause decompensation of the cardiac failure. However, there was no biochemical evidence of myocardial necrosis (normal CK and Troponin T). The ECG did not show evidence of acute pericarditis. The lack of raised inflammatory markers makes the diagnosis of chest infection unlikely. The most likely explanation is water retention due to the use of indomethacin, a non-steroidal anti-inflammatory drug (NSAID). NSAIDs work by inhibition of cyclo-oxygenase enzyme (COX) of which are two types:

- COX-1 has many "physiologic" actions
- COX-2 has "inflammatory" effects

Inhibition of COX-2 in the kidney results in decreased renal blood flow and glomerular filtration rate, thereby leading to water retention.

Drugs causing water retention

- Corticosteroids
- Mineralocorticoids (e.g. fludrocortisone)
- Sex hormones
- NSAIDs
- Carbenoxolone
- Minoxidil
- Diazoxide
- Ciclosporin

Common side effects of NSAID

- Systemic and local NSAID's contribute to gastrointestinal damage: nausea, vomiting, diarrhoea, ulceration and bleeding.
- Pancreatitis

- Hepatitis
- Hypersensitivity reactions: rash, angio-oedema and bronchospasm
- Skin complications: rash, Stevens-Johnson syndrome, toxic epidermal necrolysis.
- Neurological: headache, dizziness, nervousness, and depression.
- Aseptic meningitis is a rare side effect.
- Fluid retention and precipitation of heart failure
- Renal impairment particularly in the elderly
- Renal papillary necrosis (rare)
- Interstitial nephritis (rare)
- Hyponatraemia
- Blood dyscrasias

Precautionary advice

- The NSAID should be used with caution in patients with renal diseases and heart failure.
- In patients at risk of duodenal or gastric ulceration, use either a selective COX–2 inhibitor, or co-prescribe a NSAID with a gastroprotective agent such proton pump inhibitor or misoprostol. The latter two provide protection against both duodenal and gastric ulceration. H-2 antagonists protect against duodenal ulceration when given in combination with NSAIDs.

Case 75

Tardive Dyskinesia

A 72-year-old man was seen in the OPD with a two weeks history of confusion and wandering at night. The wife first noticed his forgetfulness over one year ago. His mini-mental state examination revealed a score of 14/30. The CT brain showed generalised cerebral atrophy. The blood count, electrolytes, liver function, vitamin B12, folate, and glucose were all normal. The diagnosis of Alzheimer's disease was made and he was commenced on Aricept (Donepezil) 5 mg od and risperidone 0.5 mg bd. The patient's behaviour gradually settled on these medications. The dose of donepezil was increased to 10 mg od. At three months follow-up there was no night-time wandering. However, the wife was concerned about his involuntary lip smacking and tongue protrusions that have appeared over the last three weeks.

What is the most likely explanation?

A. Dystonic reaction
B. Akathisia
C. Tardive dyskinesia
D. Parkinsonism
E. Myoclonic jerks

Diagnosis (C)

DISCUSSION

Major tranquilizers are commonly used in the elderly. Compared to younger patients, elderly patients are more sensitive to their side effects. This patient has tardive dyskinesia.

Side effects of phenothiazines and major tranquilizers

Neurological	• Extrapyramidal side effects • Neuroleptic malignant syndrome • Drowsiness • Agitation • Convulsions • Insomnia • Confusion
Autonomic nervous system	• Interference with temperature regulation • Anti-muscarinic symptoms (e.g. dry mouth, constipation, difficulty in micturition, and blurred vision)
Cardiovascular	• Hypotension • Tachycardia • Arrhythmia
Endocrine	• Galactorrhoea • Gynaecomastia • Impotence • Weight gain
Others	• Gastrointestinal disturbances • Blood dyscrasia • Photosensitivity • Pigmentation of the skin, cornea, conjunctiva and retina • Cholestatic jaundice

Extrapyramidal side effects

- Tardive dyskinesia is a dystonic-dyskinetic syndrome often involving the face (lip-smacking, protruding tongue) and is usually a side effect of medium to long-term treatment with antipsychotics. Tardive dyskinesia can be exacerbated by stopping antipsychotic treatment.
- Parkinsonism. These extrapyramidal side effects, such as bradykinesia and tremor, resemble Parkinson's disease.
- Akathisia is a feeling of physical restlessness and inability to keep still and often involve the feet. This may be confused with agitation and incorrectly treated with higher doses of antipsychotics that inevitably will worsen the symptoms.
- Dystonias are abnormal involuntary movement that may be painful and can appear after only a few doses.

Atypical antipsychotic drugs: effects on mortality and stroke

Atypical antipsychotic drugs should be used with caution especially in elderly patients with dementia, because of their extrapyramidal side effects and in light of recent reports on increased mortality. In elderly patients with dementia, increased cardiovascular morbidity and mortality is reported with thioridazine, olanzapine and risperidone.

Thioridazine

Thioridazine (Melleril) has been shown to prolong the QT interval in a dose related manner. Drugs that prolong QT interval have been associated with life-threatening arrhythmias including torsades-de-pointes arrhythmias and sudden death. Therefore, thioridazine should be reserved for the treatment of schizophrenic patients who fail to show an acceptable response to adequate courses of other antipsychotic drugs. The use of thioridazine in elderly patients with dementia has been discontinued.

Olanzapine and Risperidone

The report by the Committee on the Safety of Medicines (CSM) of the United Kingdom on atypical antipsychotic drugs and increased stroke risk (CEM/CMO/2004/1) is summarized below:

- Although no atypical antipsychotic drug is licensed for the treatment of behavioural disturbance in dementia, they are quite frequently used for this purpose and manufacturers have conducted clinical trials in this indication. The Committee has reviewed the available data from trials of risperidone and olanzapine and considered other relevant evidence.
- Evidence reviewed by the Committee on Safety of Medicines indicates an increased risk of stroke, which particularly applies when these drugs (olanzapine and risperidone) are used by elderly patients with dementia.
- Risperidone is the most extensively studied drug in this context and a meta-analysis of randomized placebo-controlled clinical trials in elderly patients with dementia has shown that, compared with placebo, the risk of stroke with risperidone was approximately three times higher.
- A pooled analysis of randomized placebo-controlled clinical trials of olanzapine in elderly patients with dementia has

shown *a similar increased risk of stroke and a 2-fold increase in all-cause mortality*. The mechanism by which these drugs are associated with stroke is unclear. Although some patients with dementia may have underlying vascular disease, the risk is not confined to this group. Although most of the evidence causing concern comes from patients with dementia, the risk may not be confined to use in this indication and should be considered relevant to any patient with a history of cerebrovascular disease or relevant risk factors.

The recommendations of the CSM

- Risperidone or olanzapine should not be used for the treatment of behavioural symptoms of dementia.
- Use of risperidone for the management of acute psychotic conditions in elderly patients who also have dementia should be limited to short-term and should be under specialist advice (olanzapine is not licensed for management of acute psychoses).
- Prescribers should consider carefully the risk of cerebrovascular events before treating any patient with a previous history of stroke or transient ischaemic attack. Consideration should also be given to other risk factors for cerebrovascular disease including hypertension, diabetes, current smoking and atrial fibrillation.
- Although there is presently insufficient evidence to include other antipsychotics in these recommendations, prescribers should bear in mind that a risk of stroke cannot be excluded, pending the availability of further evidence. Studies to investigate this are being initiated.
- Patients with dementia who are currently treated with an atypical antipsychotic drug should have their treatment reviewed. Many patients with dementia who are disturbed may be managed without medicines.

LINKS WITH BOOK ONE

1. Case 22, page 60. Lewy Body Dementia (discussion on types of dementia, mental test scores, and acetylcholinesterase inhibitors in Alzheimer's disease).
2. Case 66, page 213. Acute confusional state and incidentaloma (discussion on causes of acute confusional state).
3. Case 81, page 270. Neuroleptic malignant syndrome.

Case 76

Atrial Fibrillation

A man brought his 82-year-old wife to the A and E with symptoms of increasing confusion over the last two days. She was known to have Alzheimer's disease and recurrent falls. On examination, she was breathless and there were fine crackles in both lung bases. The heart rate was irregular at 154 bpm with blood pressure 180/110 mmHg. The ECG showed atrial fibrillation with a fast ventricular rate and widespread ST segment depression. Levels of CK and troponin T were normal. The patient was given oxygen, furosemide and digoxin. Two hours later, she was less breathless, but still in atrial fibrillation with an apex heart rate was 80-90 bpm.

What is the most appropriate option in this patient for the reduction of thrombo-embolism?

A. Warfarin
B. Aspirin
C. Cardioversion
D. Dipyridamole
E. Sulphinpyrazone

Answer (B)

DISCUSSION

This patient is not suitable for warfarin therapy because of recurrent falls and severe dementia. The other prophylactic measure against thromboembolism is antiplatelet therapy. Aspirin reduces the risk of thromboembolism by about 20 per cent in patients with atrial fibrillation. Dipyridamole and sulphinpyrazone are ineffective.

Lone atrial fibrillation

Lone AF is not associated with clinical, echocardiographic or electrocardiographic evidence of cardiopulmonary disease. These patients are usually young (under 60 years) and have low risk of thromboembolism and mortality. Therefore, prophylactic anti-thrombotic treatment is not required. As the age advances, these patients may develop other risk factors, which will warrant prophylactic antiplatelet or anti-coagulant therapy.

Non-valvular atrial fibrillation (AF)

By convention, the term "non-valvular AF" is used when AF occurs in the absence of rheumatic mitral valve disease or a prosthetic heart valve.

Acute atrial fibrillation secondary to treatable medical conditions

Atrial fibrillation may complicate acute medical conditions including:

- Acute myocardial infarction
- Chest infection
- Acute pulmonary oedema
- Pulmonary embolism
- Cardiac surgery
- Acute pericarditis or myocarditis

In these acute situations the main therapeutic aims are:

- Restore sinus rhythm by cardioversion if the patient is not tolerating the arrhythmia i.e. hypotension, breathlessness or confusion.
- Control the ventricular rate if cardioversion is futile or contraindicated
- Short-term anticoagulant depending on the duration of arrhythmia.

Usually the atrial fibrillation is reversible when the underlying medical condition is treated or stabilised. Therefore, these patients do not require long-term anticoagulation and medications to prevent relapse of AF.

Causes of atrial fibrillation in patients attending for electrical cardioversion

In large consecutive series of patients undergoing elective DC cardioversion for AF, the following underlying conditions were found:

- Ischaemic heart disease
- Rheumatic valvular disease
- Lone AF
- Hypertension
- Cardiomyopathy
- Non-rheumatic valvular disease
- Congenital heart disease
- Treated hyperthyroidism

Patterns of atrial fibrillation

Paroxysmal AF: When AF is recurrent $\geq$ 2 times and terminate spontaneously.

Persistent AF: Persistent AF does not terminate spontaneously. It could be the first episode of AF or the culmination of recurrent episode of paroxysmal AF. *The arrhythmia is still called persistent even after successful cardioversion*

Permanent AF: When AF has been present for more than one year, it is called permanent AF.

Cardioversion for atrial fibrillation

Restoration of sinus rhythm may be done by pharmacological agents or electrical cardioversion. Both acute AF (including paroxysmal AF) and persistent AF require emergency cardioversion if they cause:

- Haemodynamic instability (e.g. hypotension)
- Acute heart failure
- Angina

Elective cardioversion has the following advantages in stable patients with persistent AF:

- Relieves symptoms
- Avoids tachyarrhythmia induced cardiomyopathy
- Improves left ventricle function
- Prevents thromboembolism

Complications of electrical cardioversion

DC electrical shock is synchronised with the R wave. The initial DC energy used for atrial flutter is 50 Joules. However for atrial fibrillation, start with 100 Joules increasing to 200 Joules and to 360 Joules when the preceding shocks fail to cardiovert. To avoid myocardial damage, the interval between two consecutive shocks should not be less than one minute.

1. *Embolism:* This can occur if pharmacological or electrical cardioversion was performed without prophylactic anticoagulation. Thromboembolism can occur in 1-7 per cent of patients. *There are reports that embolisation may occur in some patients following cardioversion despite prophylactic anticoagulation.*

2. *Arrhythmias:* Following electrical cardioversion, the following complications may arise:
   - Benign arrhythmia such as supraventricular and ventricular ectopic beats, bradycardia and transient sino-atrial pauses
   - Serious arrhythmias such as ventricular tachycardia or fibrillation are more likely if the patient has:
     a. Hypoxia
     b. Hypokalaemia
     c. Digoxin toxicity. Electrical cardioversion is contraindicated in digitalis toxicity.

3. *Myocardial injury:* Repeated DC shocks may cause myocardial necrosis.

Cardioversion for recurrent persistent atrial fibrillation

A Comparison of Rate Control and Rhythm Control in Patients with Recurrent Persistent Atrial Fibrillation (Van Gelder IC et al. NEJM 2002;347:1834-1840). In this study, the authors hypothesized that ventricular rate control was not inferior to the maintenance of sinus rhythm for the treatment of atrial fibrillation. They randomly assigned 522 patients *who had persistent atrial fibrillation after a previous electrical cardioversion to:*
- Receive treatment aimed at rate control: these patients received oral anticoagulant drugs and rate-slowing medication;
- Patients in the rhythm-control group underwent serial cardioversions and received antiarrhythmic drugs and oral anticoagulants.

The study end points were:
- Death from cardiovascular causes
- Heart failure
- Thromboembolic complications
- Bleeding
- Implantation of a pacemaker
- Severe drug adverse effects

The patients were followed up for period of 2.3 ± 0.6 years (SD) and the results were as follows:

- Thirty nine percent of the 266 patients in the rhythm-control group had sinus rhythm, as compared with 10 per cent of the 256 patients in the rate-control group.
- The primary end point was observed in 44 patients (17.2 per cent) in the rate-control group compared to 60 patients (22.6 per cent) in the rhythm-control group.
- They concluded that rate control was not inferior to rhythm control for the prevention of death and morbidity from cardiovascular causes and may be appropriate therapy in patients with a recurrence of persistent atrial fibrillation after electrical cardioversion.

Prophylactic anticoagulation for cardioversion

- If thrombi are present in the left atrium, restoration of sinus rhythm may enhance dislodging of thrombi.
- Electrical cardioversion may cause temporary left atrial and left atrial appendage (LAA) mechanical dysfunction called "myocardial stunning".
- Restoration of left atrial and LAA function after stunning may be complicated by embolisation of intra-atrial thrombi produced during the period of stunning.
- It is advisable for anticoagulation to be started with heparin in patients who need immediate cardioversion.
- A bolus dose of heparin is followed by IV infusion to keep APTT ratio at 1.5–2.0 for 2-3 days. This should be followed by oral anticoagulants for 3-4 weeks.
- In patients with acute (recent) AF of more than two days duration or of unknown duration, but who are stable and do not require immediate cardioversion, one would anticoagulate these patients with warfarin (INR 2-3) for 3-4 weeks after which cardioversion is attempted. Anticoagulation is continued for 4 weeks after the cardioversion if sinus rhythm has been restored, otherwise it is continued indefinitely with a target INR of 2-3.
- Anticoagulation for persistent AF. Anticoagulate with warfarin (INR 2-3) for 3-4 weeks and continue anticoagulation for another four weeks after successful cardioversion with restoration of sinus rhythm.

Pharmacological management atrial fibrillation

Pharmacological cardioversion: This is less effective than electrical cardioversion. The drugs that are commonly used are:

- Amiodarone
- Flecainide
- Propafenone
- Quinidine

Drugs that should not be used for cardioversion of atrial fibrillation

- Beta-blockers. The exception is esmolol as it may be effective in the cardioversion of recent onset AF, but this has not been tested in clinical trials.
- Digoxin. Not effective
- Sotalol. No proven efficacy
- Oral disopyramide

Drugs to control ventricular rate in atrial fibrillation

The target heart rate in atrial fibrillation is as follows:

- Resting heart rate: 60-80 bpm
- Exercise heart rate: 90-115 bpm

The drugs that are commonly used to control ventricular rate are:

- Beta-blockers
- Diltiazem
- Verapamil (not to be combined with beta-blocker)
- Digoxin. Some patients with atrial fibrillation show an excessive increase in heart rate with exercise, which is not controlled by digoxin even in therapeutic doses. Try adding a small dose of a beta-blocker, diltiazem or verapamil in these patients.

Drugs used to prevent paroxysmal atrial fibrillation

- Beta-blockers are especially effective in patients with lone AF and angina
- Amiodarone is the drug of choice for patients with congestive heart failure and those with structural heart diseases.
- Sotalol is not effective for cardioversion, but may be useful to prevent paroxysmal AF. *The effective dose is 80-160 mg bd.*

- Flecainide and propafenone can be safely used in those who have normal left ventricular function and no structural heart disease.
- Digoxin is useless in the prevention of paroxysmal AF.

Atrial fibrillation in Wolfe-Parkinson-White (WPW) syndrome

- Drugs that reduce conduction in the accessory pathway such as flecainide and propafenone are preferred.
- The most effective method to terminate AF in WPW is electrical cardioversion followed by radiofrequency ablation of the accessory pathway.
- Digoxin is contraindicated.
- Beta-blockers do not decrease the conduction in the accessory pathway during pre-excited periods of AF and can worsen the arrhythmia or hypotension.
- Calcium channel blocker: verapamil and diltiazem are contraindicated (same reasons as in beta-blockers).

LINKS TO BOOK ONE

1. Case 86, page 291. Atrial fibrillation with complete heart block (Discussion on warfarin versus aspirin).
2. Case 87, page 293. Atrial fibrillation.

Case 77

Poor Control of Hypertension

A 65-year-old man was referred by his GP for treatment of poorly controlled hypertension. The blood pressure readings taken at the GP surgery in the last 6 months were:

- October 2003 — 210/120 mmHg
- November 2003 — 180/104 mmHg
- January 2004 — 170/100 mmHg

His medications were bendroflumethiazide 2.5 mg od and amlodipine 10 mg od. He smoked 20 cigarettes a day and took one glass of wine with dinner. On examination, he was obese (BMI = 31), the heart was in sinus rhythm with no features of cardiac failure and the blood pressure (sitting) was 192/110 mmHg. The following results became available after his clinic appointment:

Na	130 mmol/l
K	3.8 mmol/l
Urea	7.2 mmol/ l
Creatinine	112 μmol/l
Glucose	5.2 mmol/l
LFT	normal
Urine	normal
Total cholesterol	7.8 mmol/l
ECG	LVH strain
CXR	cardiomegaly
Abdominal ultrasound	normal size kidneys, no obstructive uropathy

What is the next best therapeutic intervention?

A. Increase bendroflumethiazide to 5 mg od
B. Add hydrochlorothiazide
C. Initiate perindopril 2 mg od

D. Add minoxidil
E. Replace amlodipine with doxazosin

Answer (C)

DISCUSSION

This patient has severe hypertension with target organ damage as indicated by:

- ECG evidence of left ventricular hypertrophy
- Cardiomegaly on chest X-ray

The main therapeutic issues for this patient include:

- Optimising his anti-hypertensive medication
- Life style modification
- Lipid lowering therapy
- Aspirin therapy

Optimising anti-hypertensive medication

- Increasing the dose of bendroflumethiazide to 5 mg will not increase its anti-hypertensive effect, but increase the side effects. Likewise, the addition of another diuretic will lead to an increase in side effects.
- Minoxidil is not a third line therapeutic agent in hypertension.
- Doxazosin is not an ideal option. The only compelling indication is the presence of benign hypertrophy of prostate with hypertension. Furthermore, the ALLHAT trial showed that doxazosin as a primary treatment for hypertension was inferior to thiazides, amlodipine and lisinopril.
- The addition of an ACE inhibitor will be the ideal therapy in this patient.

Life style modification

- Maintain normal weight (body mass index = 20-25 kg/m^2).
- Reduce salt intake to < 100 mmol/day (< 6g NaCl or < 2.4 g Na^+/day).
- Limit alcohol consumption to < 3 units/day for men (< 2 units/day for women).
- Engage in regular aerobic physical exercise (i.e. brisk walking is better than weightlifting) for > 30 minutes a day, ideally on most of days of the week but at least on three days of the week.

- Consume at least five portions of fresh fruit and vegetables each day
- Reduce the intake of total and saturated fat.
- Stop smoking

The beneficial effects of stopping smoking

- Giving up smoking should be encouraged. This can be supported by nicotine replacement therapy and attendance at smoking cessation clinics.
- Both pulse rate and blood pressure may fall within 60 minutes.
- Within 8 hours of cessation of smoking arterial oxygen levels improve
- About 24 hours later carbon monoxide is eliminated from the body and the lungs start to clear out mucus and smoking related debris.
- Beneficial effects on chronic bronchitis are observed after 3 to 9 months.
- After five years the heart attack risk falls to about one half that of a smoker.
- After ten years the lung cancer risk falls to about one half that of a smoker.

Table 77.1: The beneficial effects from a 10 kg loss in weight

Mortality	• Total mortality fall by 20-25% • Diabetes related death fall by 30-40% • Obesity related cancer death fall by 40-50%
Blood Pressure	• Systolic and diastolic fall by 10 mmHg
Diabetes	• Risk of developing diabetes reduced by > 50% • Fasting blood glucose fall by 30-50% • HbA1c fall by 15%
Lipids	• Total cholesterol fall by 10% • LDL cholesterol fall by 15% • Triglycerides fall by 30% • HDL increase by 8%

When to start anti hypertensive therapy

1. BP systolic 140-159 mmHg and or diastolic BP 90-99 mmHg, if
   a. Target organ damage
   b. Diabetes mellitus

c. Estimated 10-year risk of cardiovascular diseases of ≥ 20 per cent despite life style advice

2. Sustained grade 2 hypertension ≥ 160/100 mmHg

Note: BP should be checked at least every five years until the age of 80 years. Individuals with BP of high normal i.e. 130-139/85-89 mmHg should have their BP checked every year and advised on life style changes.

High risk patients

1. Type 2 diabetes. The majority are > 50 years or whose condition has been diagnosed ≥ 10 years. These patients have a risk of cardiovascular disease equivalent to people who have had a myocardial infarction. They should receive secondary prevention.
2. High risk (> 20% in 5 years) include:
   i. Symptomatic cardiovascular diseases including:
      1. Angina
      2. Myocardial infarction
      3. Congestive heart failure
      4. Transient ischaemic attacks and stroke
      5. Peripheral vascular disease

   ii. Electrocardiographic left ventricular hypertrophy

For other patients one should refer to new risk prediction chart on the website of British Hypertension Society (http://www.bhsoc.org/).

Choice of Antihypertensive drugs

The British Hypertension Society (2004) has adopted a simple approach based on:

- High renin hypertension - younger patients < 55 years
- Low renin hypertension - older patients and black population

In the high renin group, it is better to initiate therapy with A or B drugs as they attenuate the angiotensin-renin system as follows:

A = Angiotensin converting enzyme inhibitor (ACEI), *or* Angiotensin receptor antagonist or blocker (ARB)

B = Beta-blocker

In the low renin group, it is better to start with C *or* D group.

C = Calcium channel blocker

D = Diuretic

Although poor compliance is a major factor for poorly controlled hypertension, monotherapy is a major factor preventing the achievement of target blood pressure in patients with hypertension. When one drug is not sufficient to control blood pressure, one option is to substitute it with another drug from a different class. However, the addition of another drug is more likely to achieve the target blood pressure, which inevitably leads to polypharmacy. The logical combinations as recommended by the BHS are:

- (A or B) + C *or* D
- (A or B) + C *and* D
- If three drugs are not effective, the following options are advised by the British Society:
  a. A + B + C + D *or*
  b. Addition of an alpha-blocker or low dose spironolactone to the triple therapy i.e. when beta-blocker is contraindicated

The use of drugs in specific classes due to compelling indications

- Beta-blocker for angina or patients post myocardial infarction
- Doxazosin for patients with hypertension and prostatic enlargement
- ARB's for patients who develop cough due to ACE-I

'Since this book has been written, the results of the ASCOT Trial have been published which had revealed that combination of amlodipine and ACEI was superior to the combination of atenolol and thiazide diuretic. Accordingly the BHS is revisiting its 2004 guidelines.'

Blood pressure targets

- Patients with diabetes, renal impairment or established cardiovascular diseases < 130/80 mmHg
- Otherwise < 140/85 mmHg

Follow up of patients

- Frequency of follow-up visits will depend on the severity of hypertension, side effects from drugs and co-morbidity.
- For stable and uncomplicated patients, six monthly follow up may be sufficient.
- Blood pressure is measured in sitting position.

- However, standing blood pressure measurement is useful in elderly and diabetic patients (danger of postural hypotension).
- Weight and body mass index.
- Urine for protein (annually) but in practice urinalysis is done at every clinic visit.
- Aspects of drug therapy: side effects, compliance.
- Search for complications of hypertension

Aspirin in hypertension

Aspirin 75 mg/day used if:

- Age ≥ 50 years
- Blood pressure controlled (≤ 150/90 mmHg)
- Target organ damage, diabetes mellitus or cardiovascular disease risk ≥ 20 percent over 10 years.

Hyperlipidaemia and hypertension

Primary prevention: patients who have hypertension but without diabetes mellitus and cardiovascular diseases. In these patients, hypercholesterolaemia (LDL cholesterol ≥ 3.5 mmol/litre) is treated with a statin provided that:

- Patients < 80 years
- Cardiovascular disease risk ≥ 20 percent over 10 years

Secondary prevention: patients with hypertension who have diabetes mellitus or cardiovascular diseases. These patients need a statin if:

- They are aged up to at least 80 years
- LDL cholesterol ≥ 3.5 mmol/litre

In both primary and secondary hypertension, the target cholesterol reductions are as follows: reduction of total cholesterol (TC) by 25 per cent or LDL by 30 per cent or TC reach < 4.0 mmol/litre or LDL < 2.0 mmol/litre. Acceptable targets are:

- TC < 5.0 mmol/litre
- LDL < 3.0 mmol/litre
- Reduction of TC by 25 per cent and LDL by 30 per cent

Grades of hypertension

The British Hypertension Society guideline (2004) for the classification and grading of hypertension is shown in the Table 77.2.

Table 77.2: British Hypertension Society classification of blood pressure levels

Category	*Systolic BP (mmHg)*	*Diastolic BP (mmHg)*
Optimal	< 120	< 80
Normal	< 130	< 85
High normal	130-139	85-89
Hypertension		
Grade 1 (mild)	140-159	90-99
Grade 2 (moderate)	160-179	100-109
Grade 3 (severe)	≥ 180	≥ 110
Isolated systolic hypertension		
Grade 1	140-159	< 90
Grade 2	≥ 160	< 90

This classification equates with those of the European Society of Hypertension and the World Health Organization-International Society of Hypertension and is based on clinic blood pressure and not values obtained from ambulatory blood pressure measurement.

Threshold blood pressure levels for the diagnosis of hypertension using self/home monitoring are greater than 135/85 mm Hg. For ambulatory monitoring 24 hour values are greater than 125/80 mm Hg. If systolic blood pressure and diastolic blood pressure fall into different categories the higher value should be taken for classification.

Potential indications for the use of ambulatory blood pressure monitoring

- Unusual variability of blood pressure
- Possible white coat hypertension
- Informing equivocal treatment decisions
- Evaluation of nocturnal hypertension
- Evaluation of drug resistant hypertension
- Determining the efficacy of drug treatment over 24 hours
- Diagnosis and treatment of hypertension in pregnancy
- Evaluation of symptomatic hypotension

Case 78

Digoxin Toxicity

A 75-year-old lady presented to the A and E department with a 3-day history of nausea and vomiting, but there was no haematemesis, abdominal pain or bowel disturbance. She was a known hypertensive and has atrial fibrillation. Her medications were digoxin 250 mcg od, bendroflumethiazide 2.5 mg od and aspirin 75 mg od. The apex heart rate was irregular at 64 bpm and blood pressure 152/58 mmHg. There was an ejection systolic murmur at the left sternal edge, a clear chest and mild epigastric tenderness, but no ankle oedema. Rectal examination was normal. The ECG showed atrial fibrillation with sagging ST-segment depression in the precordial leads. The chest X-ray did not show any free gas under the diaphragms and the abdominal X-ray did not show any fluid levels.

Hb	13.2 g/dl
WBC	7.4 x 10^9/l
Platelets	210 x 10^9/l
Na	142 mmol/l
K	3.1 mmol/l
Urea	11.0 mmol/l
CRP	< 10 mg/l
Creatinine	150 µmol/l
LFT	normal
Glucose	7.1 mmol/l

What is the next most useful investigation?

A. Gastroscopy
B. Ultrasound scan of abdomen
C. CT abdomen

D. Serum digoxin levels
E. Diagnostic laporotomy

Answer (D)

DISCUSSION

Digoxin Toxicity

Digoxin is a cardiac glycoside with positive inotropic effects. Inhibition of myocardial Na^+-K^+-ATP-ase enzyme by digoxin leads to an increase in intracellular sodium and calcium concentrations. Greater availability of calcium enhances actin-myosin interaction and produces increased myocardial contractility. The other actions of digoxin are:

- Increased baroreceptor responsiveness and vagal stimulation
- Reduced sympathetic output

The half-life of digoxin is about 36 hours and once in the circulation, it is partly bound to plasma proteins. About 80 per cent of digoxin is excreted unchanged in the urine. The loading dose of digoxin is 0.5 to 1.0 mg and the maintenance dose is 125 to 250 mcg a day. In children and the elderly, the maintenance dose is lower at around 62.5 mcg a day. Plasma levels are used to detect toxicity and the trough levels (just before the next dose) should be in the therapeutic range of 1.0 to 2.6 nmol/l (equivalent to 0.8 to 2.0 ng/ml). However, patients could have features of digoxin toxicity in the presence of therapeutic plasma levels. The latter can occur in the patients with hypokalaemia and hypomagnesaemia. Use digoxin with caution in patients with hyperthyroidism as they may not respond well to digoxin but can develop toxicity if the dosage is increased.

Precipitating factors for digoxin toxicity

- Hypokalaemia
- Hypomagnesaemia
- Renal failure
- Old age
- Hyperthyroidism

Clinical presentation of digoxin toxicity

- Nausea and vomiting
- Altered vision (xanthopsia)

- Confusion
- Arrhythmias
- Conduction defects
- Digoxin level > 2.6 nmol/l (or > 2.0 ng/ml)

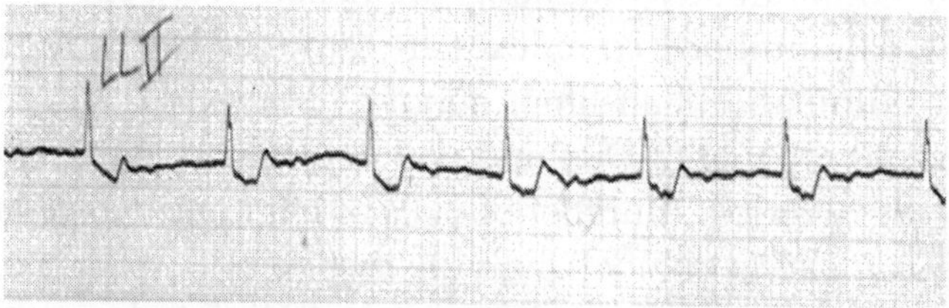

Figure 78.1: Atrial fibrillation with sagging ST-segment depression due to digoxin treatment.
Note: ST-segment depression in someone taking digoxin does not indicate toxicity.

Treatment of Digoxin Toxicity

- Stop digoxin.
- Correction of hypokalaemia and hypomagnesaemia. *Note*: Hyperkalaemia is a feature of digoxin toxicity, as Na^+-K^+-ATP-ase ejects potassium out of cells and is resistant to glucose-insulin (see indication for Digibind below).
- Treatment of conduction defects and arrhythmias.
  - Phenytoin, magnesium and lignocaine for tachyarrhythmias
  - Pacing for bradyarrhythmias and high grade AV block (transcutaneous pacing is safer, as transvenous pacing wire may precipitate serious tachyarrhythmias).
  - DC cardioversion for tachyarrythmias is potentially dangerous in digoxin toxicity as there is a risk of refractory VT or VF. If DC cardioversion is unavoidable, start with 25 Joules. DC cardioversion thought to be safe if serum digoxin level is < 2.6 nmol/l (or < 2 ng/ml).
  - Digoxin antibody is useful in serious overdose (see below).

Digoxin-specific Antibody Fragments (Digibind)

- Indications for Digibind therapy are:
  - Life threatening arrhythmias (VF, VT).
  - Bradycardia, high grade AV block, asystole.
  - Large overdose: 10 mg of digoxin in adults.

  - Serum digoxin level > 7.8 nmol/l (> 6 ng/ml) in chronic poisoning.
  - Hyperkalaemia (> 5.5 mmol/l) that is resistant to glucose-insulin.
- Digoxin antibody fragments are raised in sheep.
- Digoxin-antibody complexes are removed by the kidneys and the elimination half-life is about 15 hours.
- One 40 mg vial of Digibind will neutralise 0.6 mg of digoxin.
- Acute overdose: number of vials of Digibind = *ingested dose of digoxin tablets (mg)* × 0.8 divide by 0.6.
- Chronic poisoning: number of vials of Digibind = *serum digoxin level (measured in nmol/l)* x body weight (kg) divide by 130.

  or

  number of vial of Digibind = *serum digoxin level (measured in ng/ml)* x body weight (kg) divide by 100.
- Digibind is mixed with normal saline: give by IV bolus in cardiac arrest situation, or by IV infusion over 30 minutes.
- Beneficial effects of Digibind occur within 30 minutes.
- Side effects include allergic problems (e.g. urticaria), hypokalaemia, and worsening heart failure is possible.

Digibind will render digoxin levels useless, as the assay cannot distinguish between digoxin and digoxin-antibody complexes.

Case 79

Septic Abortion and DIC

A medical registrar was called by an obstetric senior medical house officer for advice on a 35-year-old lady who had not menstruated for three months. On examination, she was drowsy, hypotensive (blood pressure 85/50 mmHg) and pale. She was also tender in the lower abdomen. The uterus was bulky and the cervical os was open with evidence of bleeding.

Hb	7.0 g/dl
WBC	21 x 10^9/l (neutrophils 78)
Platelets	52 x 10^9/l

What is the diagnosis?

A. Septic abortion
B. Disseminated intravascular coagulation
C. Acute salpingitis
D. Septic abortion, septicaemia and disseminated intravascular coagulation
E. Abscess in the rectovaginal pouch

Answer (D)

DISCUSSION

She has the clinical features of abortion with septicaemia. In this context the low platelet count suggests disseminated intravascular coagulation. The essential management measures are:

- Blood cultures
- Urine cultures
- Culture of vaginal discharge
- Blood transfusion

- Intravenous antibiotics including cover for *Staphylococcus aureus* and anaerobes, e.g. IV ceftazidime, flucloxacillin and metronidazole
- Evacuation of the uterus
- Coagulation screen and FDP assay

LINKS TO BOOK ONE

1. Case 57, page 177. Disseminated intravascular coagulation.

Case 80

Herpes Zoster of the Bladder

A 74-year-old man presented with a seven-day history of pain in the buttock and difficulty in micturition. One year ago he underwent a transurethral resection of the prostate. He has been treated for angina pectoris for the past two years. He was a non-smoker and seldom drank alcohol. His only medications were isosorbide dinitrate and glyceryl trinitrate sublingual spray. On examination, he was apyrexial, heart and chest were normal. The bladder was not distended and rectal examination showed the prostate was not enlarged. There was a vesicular rash over the sacrum and the right buttock.

FBC	normal
Glucose	6.6 mmol/l
Na	138 mmol/l
K	4.6 mmol/l
Urea	8.3 mmol/l
Creatinine	118 μmol/l
Urinalysis	normal
Abdominal ultrasound	both kidneys were not enlarged and there was no evidence of obstruction.

What is the most likely diagnosis?

A. Herpes zoster
B. Herpes simplex
C. Herpangina
D. Drug eruption
E. Dermatitis herpetiformis

Answer (A)

DISCUSSION

This patient had severe pain in the right buttock with difficulty in micturition. This is an alarming combination of symptoms and should always raise the suspicion of serious neurological problems, such as spinal cord compression (cauda equina syndrome) or radiculopathy. However, the appearance of a herpetic vesicular rash that was confined to the right buttock solved this diagnostic riddle. The urinary symptoms were due to irritation of the sacral nerves that innervate the detrusor muscle of the bladder.

Case 81

Leptospirosis

A 28-year-old sewage worker presented with a 7 days history of flu-like symptoms and passed dark urine. He denied alcohol or drug abuse and was not on any regular medications. Clinically, he was mildly jaundiced and tender in the right hypochondrium. The chest was clear and heart sounds normal.

Hb	12.5 g/dl
WBC	$19.5 \times 10^9/l$
Platelets	$135 \times 10^9/l$
Bilirubin	78 μmol/l
AST	966 U/l
ALT	1850 U/l
Total protein	68 g/l
ALP	495 U/l
Albumin	42 g/l
γ-GT	358 U/l

The most likely diagnosis is:

A. Brucellosis
B. Leptospirosis
C. Legionellosis
D. Amoebiasis
E. Fulminant tuberculosis

Answer (B)

DISCUSSION

Leptospirosis

A reservoir of leptospiral infection exists in some animals. The organism is excreted in their urine and enters the human host through skin abrasions or intact mucous membranes.

Common serotypes

1. *Leptospira icterohaemorrhagiae* (rodents)
2. *L. canicola* (dogs)
3. *L. pomona, L. interrogans* (cattle, pigs)

At risk groups

1. Occupational exposure: sewer workers, veterinarians, farmers, abattoir workers
2. Recreational exposure: water sport enthusiasts

Incubation period

1. Usually 7-12 days (range 2-20 days)

Clinical features

1. First stage (leptosepticaemic phase) 4-7 days. Flu-like symptoms, including fever, myalgia, and headache, are followed by an afebrile interval of 1-3 days.
2. Second stage (immune or leptospiruric phase) 30 days or more. Fever recurs, serum antibodies appear, and *Leptospira* is excreted in the urine.
3. 50 per cent of patients have meningitis.
4. 5 to 10 per cent developed a severe illness with deep jaundice, renal failure, respiratory failure, and bleeding diathesis. Other features include haemolysis, rhabdomyolysis, and cardiac failure.
5. 90 per cent of patients do not develop jaundice and have a mild disease course.
6. Jaundice appears to be more common with *L. icterohaemorrhagiae*.

Laboratory findings

1. Mild thrombocytopenia in 50 per cent of patients
2. Marked leucocytosis (this is usually not a feature of viral hepatitis)
3. Prolonged prothrombin time
4. Uraemia and jaundice
5. Raised alkaline phosphatase. Serum transaminase may be only modestly elevated in some patients.
6. Raised CK

Diagnosis

1. *Leptospira* can be isolated from the blood and CSF during the first week.
2. *Leptospira* is excreted in the urine from the second week onwards.
3. IgM anti-leptospiral antibodies appear during the second week.

Treatment

1. Supportive therapy for multi-organ failure
2. IV benzylpenicillin. Alternatives are erythromycin and doxycycline.

Prognosis

1. Most patients recovery fully
2. Renal and hepatic dysfunction usually resolve completely
3. The mortality in severe icteric disease is > 20 percent

Prevention

1. Public health measures e.g. avoid contact with contaminated water; vaccinate high-risk waters and domestic livestock. Vaccinated dogs can still acquire leptospiral infection and excrete this organism in their urine.
2. Doxycycline (200 mg once a week) is only recommended for short term protection; it may also prevent disease in those exposed to *Leptospira* contaminated urine.

Case 82

Neisseria Meningitidis

An 18-year-old student nurse was brought to the A and E by her boyfriend. She had been unwell over the last 24 hours with pyrexia, aches and pains, headache and lethargy. On examination, the heart rate was regular at 112 bpm, temperature was 38.5° Celsius (axilla), and blood pressure 106/70 mmHg. There was a widespread petechial rash on the trunk and extremities. Neck movements were uncomfortable. She was alert with no focal neurological signs. Urinalysis showed WBC ++, protein + and blood +.

What is the most likely organism causing her illness?

A. Echo virus
B. Epstein-Barr virus
C. *Haemophilus influenzae*
D. *Escherichia coli*
E. *Neisseria meningitidis*

Answer (E)

DISCUSSION

Neisseria Meningitidis

1. *Neisseria meningitidis* is a gram-negative *Diplococcus*, located normally in the mucosa of the upper respiratory tract. It spreads from person to person by droplets and direct mucosal contact. Only a small proportion of those colonized with virulent strains will develop invasive disease.
2. Patients develop invasive disease 2 to 4 days after acquiring the virulent strain, but some may remain asymptomatic for several weeks before invasion begins.

3. There are 12 different serogroups with serogroups A, B and C accounting for more than 90 percent of all isolates.
4. The most common age group to be infected is children under 4 years of age, and another smaller peak is aged 13 to 20 years.
5. Predisposing factors for invasive disease are lack of protective antibodies, defects in the complement system, and influenza A infection.
6. In temperate climates most cases occur during the winter and early spring.

Specific investigations

1. Blood culture (10 ml for adults)
2. Swabs from the nasopharynx and the tonsils
3. Visualization of *N meningitidis*. Intra and extracellular diplococci can be observed in the cerebrospinal fluid and biopsies of haemorrhagic skin lesions using Gram stain.
4. Polymerase chain reaction can detect meningococci in the cerebrospinal fluid and blood.

Clinical presentation

1. Meningitis without shock
2. Shock without meningitis
3. Meningitis and shock
4. Meningococcaemia without shock or meningitis
5. Other manifestations

Meningitis without shock

The onset is insidious with symptoms and signs of meningism dominating the clinical picture. The diagnosis is supported by the presence of petechiae and symptoms of meningitis. Haemorrhagic lesions occur in > 70 per cent of all cases. They appear as red or bluish petechiae and indicate meningococcaemia. In fulminant meningococcal septicaemia the lesions are larger ecchymoses. Haemorrhagic lesions also occur in the conjunctivae. The CSF shows a marked leucocytosis ($>100 \times 10^6$ leucocytes/l), increased protein, decreased glucose, and gram-negative diplococci on microscopy.

Shock without meningitis

This is also known as fulminant meningococcal septicaemia (or Waterhouse–Friderichsen syndrome). The onset is characteristically rapid with symptoms and signs developing within hours. Circulatory collapse dominates the clinical picture and death is usually within 48 hours. Other features include: severe coagulopathy (resulting in extensive skin haemorrhage and thrombosis of the extremities); and impaired renal, adrenal, and pulmonary function (adult respiratory distress syndrome). *Lumbar puncture should be avoided in view of the bleeding diathesis.*

Splenectomised persons are prone to overwhelming infection with *Neisseria meningitidis, Streptococcus pneumoniae, Haemophilus influenzae, Streptococcus pyogenes* and viral haemorrhagic fevers.

Meningitis and shock

This is a combination of clinical meningitis and septicaemia

Meningococcaemia without shock or meningitis

Without treatment these patients may develop meningitis or fulminant shock.

Other manifestations

1. Transient benign meningococcaemia
2. Subacute meningococcaemia
3. Chronic meningococcaemia
4. Pericarditis
5. Arthritis involving one, or rarely, several large joints
6. Arthritis induced by immune complexes - one or several large joints
7. Cutaneous vasculitis
8. Ocular infections: episcleritis, conjunctivitis, or panophthalmitis
9. Pneumonia

Clinical picture	*Case fatality rate*
Meningitis without shock	< 5 per cent
Shock without meningitis	30 to 50 per cent

Treatment

The primary aim is to stop the rapid proliferation of meningococci in the circulation. Pre-hospital antibiotic treatment (i.e. intravenous benzylpenicillin) is commenced in suspected cases.

Antibiotic treatment

Antibiotic treatment should be initiated promptly. The choice includes: benzylpenicillin, chloramphenicol, cefotaxime and ceftriaxone, which are bactericidal to *N meningitidis*. Benzylpenicillin remains the drug of choice, but enters the CSF relatively poorly and hence, high doses are necessary. Chloramphenicol is a good alternative in patients who are hypersensitive to penicillin. Cefotaxime and ceftriaxone both penetrate the blood-brain barrier better than benzylpenicillin.

Supportive treatment

1. Volume replacement, inotropic and renal support in the acute phase
2. Corticosteroids are not recommended routinely unless a deficiency is documented

Sequelae

1. Meningitis: neurogenic deafness occurs in 1 to 10 per cent of these patients and is irreversible.
2. Shock and coagulopathy results in gangrene of the extremities, necrotic skin lesions, renal failure, and adrenal insufficiency.
3. Acute respiratory distress syndrome may lead to pulmonary fibrosis.

Vaccination

1. The serogroup A polysaccharide vaccine is immunogenic from 6 months of age. Infants of less than 24 months should be given two doses 1-month apart, whereas those above two years should be given one dose.
2. The serogroup C polysaccharide vaccine induces a normal immune response above 18 months of age and is given as a single dose.

Indications for vaccination with A or C polysaccharide vaccine

1. Close contacts of an index case
2. Travelers to high-risk areas
3. Military recruits
4. Persons with asplenia

5. Alcoholics
6. Deficiencies in the late complement components and properdin
7. Outbreak. An outbreak can be defined in the following ways:
    - If two or more individuals are attacked by the same strain in a class or day centre.
    - The attack rate exceeds 10 cases per 100,000 of the population for 3 months.
    - The attack exceeds 1 case per 1,000 with 3 or more cases in a closed group setting.

Secondary prophylaxis

1. Close contacts should be treated with rifampicin in a dose of 10 mg/kg (maximum dose 600 mg every 12 h for 48 h)
2. 500 mg of ciprofloxacin or 400 mg of ofloxacin as a single dose.
3. Pregnant women should receive 250 mg, and children of less than 12 years 125 mg, of ceftriaxone as one intramuscular injection.

Case 83

Toxic Shock Syndrome

A 34-year-old teacher was brought to the A and E by her boyfriend. She lived alone and has two cats. She has been unwell over the last two days with fever, muscle aches, confusion and diarrhoea. She has been menstruating and using tampons. Six months earlier she had a similar episode that responded to treatment. There has been no recent travel abroad. Ten years ago she was treated for thyrotoxicosis with anti-thyroid medication and subsequently underwent thyroidectomy. She was currently on thyroxine 100 μg od. On examination, there was a diffuse skin rash. She was disorientated, but there were no signs of meningeal irritation. The temperature was 38.2° Celsius, heart rate regular at 128 bpm and blood pressure 80/40 mmHg.

What is the most likely diagnosis?

A. Viral gastroenteritis
B. *Campylobacter enteritis*
C. Thyrotoxic crisis
D. Carcinoid syndrome
E. Toxic shock syndrome

Answer (E)

DISCUSSION

Toxic Shock Syndrome (TSS)

Toxic shock syndrome (TSS) is characterized by fever, rash, hypotension and multi-organ involvement (cardiovascular, renal, skin, mucosa, gastrointestinal, musculoskeletal, hepatic, haematological, and central nervous systems). The TSS is a toxin-mediated disease. The toxins activate production of tumor necrosis factor, interleukin-1, M protein, and gamma-interferon. Usually the syndrome is due to toxins of *Staphylococcus aureus* as shown in the Table 83.1. However, a toxic shock like syndrome has been described in association with and Group A beta-hemolytic streptococci (*Streptococcus pyogenes*).

Table 83.1: The bacteria and their toxins causing toxic shock syndrome

Bacteria	*Toxin*
Staphylococcus aureus	Endotoxin toxic shock syndrome toxin-1 (TSST-1)
Streptococcus pyogenes	Exotoxin A and exotoxin B

Predisposing factors

The TSS has been typically associated with tampon use in healthy menstruating women. The disease is now known to also exist in men, neonates, and non-menstruating women. The predominant risk factors include:

1. Use of super-absorbent tampons
2. Postoperative wound infection
3. Postpartum toxic shock
4. Nasal packing
5. Common bacterial infections
6. Viral infection with influenza A or varicella
7. Diabetes mellitus
8. Infection with HIV
9. Chronic cardiac and pulmonary disease

Clinical features

1. A prodromal period of 2 to 3 days is followed by systemic symptoms such as nausea, vomiting, watery diarrhoea, myalgias, arthralgias and headache.
2. Confusion sets in and the patient becomes pyrexial and hypotensive.
3. Skin rash: the rash initially appears on the trunk and spreads to the arms and legs involving palms and soles. Diffuse desquamation occurs 1 to 2 weeks later
4. Multi-organ involvement: disseminated intravascular coagulation (DIC) and acute respiratory distress syndrome.
5. The absence of evidence of other infective or vasculitic conditions
6. Even with effective treatment, the mortality is around 10 per cent

The US Centre for Disease Control and Prevention (CDC) criteria for the diagnosis of staphylococcal TSS includes all the above features but the skin rash is not stated as a criterion for the diagnosis of streptococcal TSS.

Complications of TSS
1. Prolonged neuromuscular abnormalities
2. Gangrene and cyanotic extremities
3. Memory and concentration difficulties

Laboratory studies

4. FBC may reveal leucocytosis
5. Blood cultures: these are often negative as the disease is caused by toxins
6. Bacterial cultures should be taken from all infected sites including blood.
7. Coagulation studies: elevated APTT and fibrin degradation products.
8. Renal and liver enzyme abnormalities may be present
9. Serologic tests: anti-TSST-1 antibodies are usually positive in low titres. In addition, serological tests are needed to exclude other septic and vasculitic conditions.

Management

1. ITU for haemodynamic monitoring and ventilatory support
2. Fluid resuscitation and oxygen therapy
3. Antibiotic treatment (see below)
4. Tampons should be removed. Urgent surgical intervention is needed for necrotizing fasciitis and myositis.
5. Infection control precautions should be taken.
6. Drainage of any pus is an essential.
7. Recurrence is possible and hence follow up is required.

Antibiotics for TSS

1. Staphylococcal aureus is usually resistant to penicillins. Therefore, β-lactamase-resistant penicillin (flucloxacillin), or cefuroxime should be used.
2. Clindamycin halts the production of toxins and may be added to penicillins in invasive infections.

3. If the infection is hospital acquired, MRSA should be assumed as the cause and therefore the antibiotics of choice are vancomycin, teicoplanin and linezolid.
4. Community-acquired infections in patients with penicillin allergy can be treated with intravenous erythromycin or clarithromycin.

Case 84

Herpes Genitalis

A 21-year-old college student attended her General Practitioner for painful lesions on the genitalia. She had recently visited Greece with a group of her girlfriends for a one week holiday and engaged in unprotected sex. On examination, she had a low-grade temperature of 37.8° Celsius and there were multiple blisters on the vulva with many other shallow ulcers. Vaginal examination was painful due to multiple tender shallow ulcers. There were no oral or conjunctival lesions. Urinalysis showed blood +, WBC + and protein +. The General Practitioner requested an MSU and obtained swabs from the ulcers for bacteriological tests.

What is the most appropriate treatment?

A. High dose oral penicillin
B. Topical clotrimazole
C. Intravenous immunoglobulin
D. Oral aciclovir
E. Parenteral ganciclovir

Answer (D)

DISCUSSION

This patient had multiple painful shallow genital ulcerations in the genital region after unprotected sexual activity. The most likely cause is genital herpes simplex.

Infective causes for genital ulceration

1. Herpes simplex: herpetic ulcer is painful, shallow, yellowish base with surrounding erythema
2. Herpes zoster

3. Primary chancre (in HIV co-infected patients, ulcer can be atypical)
4. Secondary syphilis causing mucous patches
5. Tertiary syphilis (gumma)
6. Chancroid (*Haemophilus ducreyi*): painful non-indurated ulcers
7. Lymphogranuloma venereum (*Chlamydia trachomatis*)
8. Granuloma inguinale

Non-infective causes for genital ulceration

1. Behçet's disease: painful punched out deep ulcers in contrast
2. Reiter's syndrome (Balanitis circinata)
3. Stevens Johnson syndrome
4. Trauma
5. Drug induced penile ulcers due to foscarnet without adequate rehydration

Check list for history taking from patients with sexually transmitted disease

Sexual infections can be asymptomatic; hence, sexual history is extremely important. Don't make assumptions, especially about sexuality and remember a (bisexual) person may have both male and female partners. Elicit if possible incubation period, source and geographic origin of infection, probability of transmission based on one sexual act or repeated multiple exposure, whether condoms were properly used, nature of coitus (to evaluate specimen sites), partners at high risk, risk factors for HIV, injecting drug use, commercial or industrial sex, etc.

History in relation to sexual disease

1. Urethral discharge
2. Genital ulceration
3. Urinary symptoms
4. Genital itching and swelling
5. Pruritus ani
6. Vaginal discharge
7. Rectal symptoms (diarrhoea, tenesmus, pain)
8. Systemic features (fever, rash, joint pain or arthritis)
9. Oral ulceration
10. Conjunctivitis
11. Menstrual history and contraception in females

12. Drug abuse and needle sharing
13. Previous STD
14. Recent travel
15. History of HIV and hepatitis screening

Sexual activities

1. Number of sexual partners (recent partner change in last 3-6 months)
2. Frequency of changing partners
3. Types of sexual activity (genital/genital, oral/genital, anal/genital, oral/anal)
4. Heterosexual/ homosexual/ bisexual
5. Regular sexual partner and/or casual sex
6. Use of barrier contraception/condom

Check list for physical examination of patients with sexually transmitted diseases

1. General examination with emphasis on: rash, lymphadenopathy, mouth and throat, eyes, and joints
2. Groin and pubic area: lymphadenopathy, infestation with lice or scabies
3. Male genitalia: balanitis, ulcers, condylomata, tumour, continuous discharge, vesicles, pigmentation and depigmentation, tenderness and/ or enlargement of testes and epididymis, and collect smears and swabs
4. Female genitalia:
   a. Identify infection in Bartholin glands
   b. Cervix: discharge, bleeding, ulceration
   c. Bimanual pelvic examination: adnexial tenderness, cervical tenderness, uterine motility and tenderness.
5. Rectal examination when indicated: pain and tenderness, tone of anal sphincter, prostatic signs, proctoscopy
6. Collect smears and swabs

Genital Herpes Simplex

HSV-2 classically accounts for 70 to 90 per cent of herpetic genital infections. HSV-1 accounts for the remaining 10 to 30 per cent. In recent years, HSV-1 is increasingly becoming prevalent in first attack episodes, in the UK. Occasionally patients may have both serotypes I and II. HSV in the sacral sensory nerve ganglia leads to periodic reactivation and re-infection of the skin. Frequent recurrences may indicate underlying immune suppression as in HIV infection.

Symptoms and signs

A. *Primary lesions*

1. Initial viral activity coincides with the prodromal phase (1-3 days before lesions appear) when patients may have symptoms of sacral neuralgia (shooting pains buttocks to back of legs), flu like feeling and/or just local itching and tingling. Prodromes can be identified in 70 to 80 per cent of attacks (and can be helpful in educating patients with frequent recurrences towards self initiated abortive therapy if started early in this phase).
2. Painful cluster of vesicles that may coalesce appear 4 to 7 days after contact. They develop into superficial ulcers, become crusted, and then heal in about 10 days.
3. Fever and regional lymphadenopathy often are present in primary infection.
4. Sites affected: prepuce, glans penis, and penile shaft (men); the labia, clitoris, perineum, vagina, and cervix (women); the anus and rectum (homosexual men or women who participate in rectal intercourse).

B. *Recurrences*

- Paraesthesia in the affected nerves usually precedes skin or mucosal lesions.
- Urinary hesitancy, acute retention and impotence may be a consequence.

Complications

1. Reactivation of latent infection
2. Aseptic meningitis
3. Transverse myelitis
4. Autonomic nervous system dysfunction (inability to urinate, constipation, and impotence in men)
5. Severe neuralgia involving the sacral regions
6. Joints, liver, or lung are involved in immunosuppressed or pregnant patients.

Diagnosis

1. Diagnosis is essentially clinical, but tests are useful for confirmation.
2. Tzanck test - characteristic multinucleated giant cells in Wright's-Giemsa-stained smears of cells from lesion.
3. Tissue culture or direct immunofluorescent assay from material swabbed from the base of ulcerated lesions or aspirated from a vesicle. Viral shedding from herpes lesions generally decrease after 72 hours (false negative culture). Asymptomatic cervical viral shedding is well described also.
4. HSV type specific serology - Paired serum samples, taken at 10 to 14 day interval, may show a rise in antibody titre in primary infections.

Treatment

1. Aciclovir either 200 mg po 5 times daily or 400 mg po every 8 hours.
2. Aciclovir-resistant herpes simplex: IV foscarnet 40 mg/kg every 8 to 12 hourly for 10 days.

Case 85

Cryptococcus Neoformans

A 65-year-old homosexual man presented to A and E because of confusion and abnormal behaviour. His male partner said that the patient had been complaining of headache for three days and had fallen twice but refused to attend hospital. On examination, he was pyrexial with a temperature of 38.8° C (axilla). He was dehydrated with mild neck stiffness and bilateral extensor plantar response. The chest X-ray was normal.

Hb	10.1 g/dl
WBC	$6.4 \times 10^9/l$
Platelets	$86 \times 10^9/l$

An urgent CT brain showed no mass or midline shift or ventricular dilatation.

Lumbar puncture	High opening pressure
	CSF protein 0.95 g/l
	CSF lymphocytes count $12/mm^3$
	CSF glucose 2.0 mmol/l (plasma glucose 7.2 mmol/l)
	Microscopy and India ink staining showed yeast cells, each with a clear halo.

What is the cause of his meningitis?

A. *Candida albicans*
B. *Cryptococcus neoformans*
C. *Toxoplasma gondii*
D. *Neisseria meningitidis*
E. *Streptococcus pneumoniae*

Answer (B)

DISCUSSION

Cryptococcus Neoformans

1. *Cryptococcus neoformans* is a fungal infection occurring in patients with impaired cell-mediated immunity. Cryptococcal meningitis in AIDS patients often present atypically, usually without signs of meningeal irritation.
2. Predisposing factors are: human immunodeficiency virus (HIV), lymphoma, solid organ transplantation, and corticosteroid therapy.
3. Transmission probably occurs via inhalation of the organism and leads to colonization and respiratory infection. The absence of cell-mediated response results in ineffective clearance with subsequent dissemination.

Clinical features

1. Subacute meningitis or meningoencephalitis presents as fever, headache, altered behaviour and impaired consciousness. Meningeal signs occur in only about one quarter of patients. Papilloedema and cranial nerve palsies (VI and VII) are common.
2. Other presentations:
   - Cryptococcal pneumonia
   - Skin involvement with lesions resembling molluscum contagiosum

Diagnosis

1. Cerebrospinal fluid (CSF) shows:
   a. Mildly elevated serum protein
   b. Normal or slightly low glucose
   c. Lymphocytosis
   d. India ink staining reveals yeast cells
   e. Cryptococcal antigen is detectable in the CSF
2. Positive serum cryptococcal antigen titre of greater than 1:8 is sensitive and specific for cryptococcal infection.
3. HIV antibody test should be performed after appropriate consent

Treatment

- The regime involves IV amphotericin B (0.7 mg/kg) for 2 weeks followed by fluconazole 400 mg orally for a further 8 weeks.

- Fluconazole 200 to 400 mg od can be given for 3 to 6 months in most patients with localized pulmonary disease.
- Extrapulmonary disease is generally managed in the same way as meningitis.
- All patients with cryptococcal meningitis should have the CSF pressure measured and if the pressure is high (> 25 cm of water), it should be reduced by repeated lumbar punctures or a shunt.

Suppressive treatment

- Cryptococcal meningitis in AIDS requires life-long suppressive therapy. Fluconazole and itraconazole are effective in preventing invasive cryptococcal infections in HIV-positive patients with CD4 counts less than 50 to 100 cells/ml.
- In other immunocompromised patients, suppressive treatment for 6 to 12 months may be given. Fluconazole 200 mg daily is the suppressive treatment of choice.

Human Immunodeficiency Virus

Human immunodeficiency virus type 1 (HIV-1) is a human retrovirus belonging to lentivirus family. HIV-2 is endemic to West Africa and seems to have a lower propensity to cause immunodeficiency than HIV-1 virus. There is evidence that HIV-2 virus has spread to the Indian subcontinent.

The virus has an envelope and core. The latter contains two copies of the RNA genome. The virus has many structural genes including:

- Gag encodes for nucleocapsid proteins within the core such as p24, p9 and p17.
- Pol contains genes responsible for major enzymes involved in HIV replication, namely reverse transcriptase, protease and integrase.
- Env is responsible for outer envelope proteins: gp 120 and gp 41 that are involved in the entry of HIV into cells.
- Rev gene is responsible for nuclear trafficking of HIV proteins.
- Tat, Nef, Vpr and Vpu genes are involved in the regulation of HIV life cycle.

Pathogenesis of HIV infection

HIV has a predilection for CD4 T-lymphocytes (T-helper cells) but may also affect other cells bearing the CD4 marker or receptors. The infection is facilitated by chemokines at the glycoprotein sites of the CD4 cells. If there is mutation of the chemokine genes (CCR5), entrance of HIV virus particles into the CD4 T-cells will be hindered. This may partly explain the resistance to HIV infection by some individuals.

Once the HIV virus has entered the CD4 T-cell, the enzyme reverse transcriptase allows viral RNA to be transcribed into the host cell's DNA thereby allowing viral replication in large amounts.

In the circulation, the HIV virus has a half-life of 6 hours, which means that to sustain any observed level of plasma viraemia, there must be a large turn over of viral production and elimination.

Methods of transmission of HIV infection

- Semen: vaginal and anal intercourse
- Cervical secretions
- Blood products
- Vertical transmission (mother to child), which occurs as follows:
  - In utero
  - During passage of baby in the birth canal
  - Breast-feeding increases vertical transmission by 20 per cent

In Africa, it is estimated that up to 40 per cent of children born to HIV infected mothers will become HIV positive. HAART with elective LSCS given in pregnancy can reduce vertical transmission to between 2 and 5 per cent in the UK. If HIV viral load is maximally suppressed to under 50 copies per ml and maintained in the last trimester, then normal vaginal delivery is recommended as safe.

Diagnostic Tests for HIV Infection

1. Anti gp 120 antibody (IgG antibody to envelope protein)
   - Appears after a latent period i.e. it is not positive in the early post infection period. This serological latency or window period may be up to 3 months.
   - Does not provide immunity.

- Remains positive in life and indicates infection.
- Is positive in neonates born to infected mothers (as it passes through the placenta) and only disappears at 18 months of age. Disappearance of these IgG antibodies confirm baby's negative HIV status.

2. Anti p24 antibody (IgG antibody to core protein)
   - Is positive in the early period after infection and in the asymptomatic period.
   - Tends to disappear as the disease progresses.
3. Viral p24 antigen
   - Usually detectable shortly after recent infection, but tends to disappear in 8 to 10 weeks after exposure
   - May reappear later at low levels.
4. Isolation of HIV-1 virus in culture (available in specialised centres) is not done routinely.
5. Viral load (HIV RNA)
   - Used for follow up of the progress of active infection.
   - It has both prognostic and therapeutic value.
   - Whatever assay is used (branched chain DNA, reverse transcriptase polymerase chain reaction RT-PCR, nucleic acid sequence based amplification NASBA) the results are expressed as copies of viral RNA per ml of plasma. The results given by different assays are variable but correlate with each other. Potency of anti retroviral agents are expressed as logs drop. Zidovudine typically reduces viral load by 1 log. More potent protease inhibitors e.g. Lopinavir or non-nucleotide reverse transcriptase inhibitors e.g. Efavirenz can reduce viral load by up to 2-3 logs.
   - The viral load for every patient is usually set by six months after sero-conversion and will determine long-term prognosis.
   - Patients with a viral load of > 10,000 copies per ml have a ten times higher risk of progression to AIDS over the next five years when compared to those who have < 10,000 copies per ml.
   - The viral load rises during intercurrent infections, such as following:
     - Influenza
     - Pneumocystis carinii pneumonia (PCP)
     - Tuberculosis

CD4 T-lymphocyte Counts

CD4 T-lymphocytes are helper cells while CD8 T-lymphocytes are cytotoxic cells. Memory T-cells are characterised by the expression of CD45 Ro antigen, whereas naïve T-cells express CD45 Ra antigen.

The normal CD4 T-lymphocyte count in healthy adult is 600 to 1500 cells/mm^3. In patients with HIV infection, a T-lymphocyte count below 500 cells/ mm^3 usually indicates HIV associated immunodeficiency. Counts of < 200/ mm^3 indicate the need for pneumocystis carinii (PCP) prophylaxis while < 100/ mm^3 call for *Mycobacterium avium* complex prophylaxis.

The CD4/CD8 ratio is variable among different subjects and the range is between 0.39 and 7.43. However, within any individual the ratio remains relatively constant. The ratio declines with the onset of symptomatic AIDS. Other causes for low CD4/CD8 ratio are:

- Acute viral infection
- Host versus graft disease
- Allograft rejections
- Haemophilia

Phases of HIV infection

1. Primary illness (seroconversion)
2. Latency
3. Persistent generalised lymphadenopathy (PGL)
4. Symptomatic HIV infection

Primary illness (seroconversion)

- Incubation period 2 to 8 weeks
- The exact proportion of patients who develop the primary infection is not known. However, it is recognised that those patients who have seroconversion have a very rapid course of progressive disease.
- Clinically presents as an acute febrile illness like infectious mononucleosis.
- There may be neurological complications including aseptic meningitis, encephalitis and myelopathy.
- Blood tests reveal lymphopenia, atypical lymphocytes on blood film, thrombocytopenia and abnormal LFTs
- Circulating CD4 lymphocytes may be markedly depleted and the CD4:CD8 ratio reversed

- Antibodies to HIV may be negative at this stage
- Anti-p 24 may be positive
- Circulating viral RNA level is very high

Latency phase

- Asymptomatic.
- Average duration is 10 years, but could be as long as 15 years. In some patients, the latency phase is only a few years.

Persistent generalised lymphadenopathy (PGL)

- Lymph nodes of 1 cm in diameter or less
- Mobile, firm and non-tender in character
- In more than two sites
- With or without splenomegaly

Symptomatic HIV infection (AIDS)

- Infections
- Malignancy

Case 86

Septic Arthritis

A 60-year-old retired physiotherapist was admitted with pain and swelling of the right knee of two days duration. She was pyrexial (39° Celsius), but there was no skin rash. She had no bowel, urinary or ocular symptoms. The knee was swollen, hot and tender with limited movements. No other joint was involved.

What condition needs to be excluded as a matter of urgency?

A. Septic arthritis
B. Crystal arthritis (gout and pseudogout)
C. Reactive arthritis
D. Rheumatoid arthritis
E. Vasculitis

Answer (A)

DISCUSSION

Any of the above-mentioned conditions can cause an acute mono-arthritis. It is important to exclude septic arthritis and screen for crystal arthritis, vasculitis and rheumatoid arthritis. The important investigations are:

- Blood cultures
- Joint aspiration (gram stain, culture and sensitivity, crystals, white cells)
- Full blood count
- CRP (or ESR)
- Biochemical screen including serum uric acid
- Vasculitic screen
- X-ray of the affected joints

Bacterial causes of septic arthritis

Gram positive bacteria

- *Staphylococcus aureus (50%)*
- *Streptococcus pyogenes*
- *Streptococcus viridans*
- *Streptococcus faecalis*
- *Pneumococci*

Gram-negative bacteria

- *Neisseria gonorrhoeae*
- *Neiserria meningitidis*
- *E. coli*
- *Haemophilus influenzae*
- *Proteus vulgaris*
- *Pseudomonas aeruginosa*
- *Klebsiella*

Predisposing factors for septic arthritis

- Diabetes mellitus
- Rheumatoid arthritis
- Prosthetic joints
- Immunosuppresive therapy and steroids

Case 87

Re-infection

A 32-year-old homosexual man presented to the genitourinary clinic with urethral discharge. He has been living with one partner for the past 10 years and both men had recently tested negative for HIV. He denied sexual intercourse outside this stable relationship. The urethral discharge was positive for *Neisseria gonorrhoeae* and responded well to penicillin. Two months later, he presented again with urethral discharge, which also revealed *Neisseria gonorrhoeae* sensitive to penicillin. He was otherwise well.

What is the most likely cause of the recurrent urethral discharge?

A. Re-infection from his partner through unprotected anal intercourse
B. Underlying tertiary syphilis leading to recurrence
C. Bacterial resistance to penicillin
D. Development of AIDS
E. Carrier of herpes simplex virus

Answer (A)

DISCUSSION

Causes of Urethral Discharge

- *Neisseria gonorrhoeae*
- *Chlamydia trachomatis*
- Herpes simplex
- Urethral warts
- Ureaplasma urealyticum
- *Mycoplasma*

- *Trichomonas vaginalis*
- Non-infective (physical or chemical trauma)

Note: Twenty per cent of men and 40 per cent of women with gonorrhoea have coexisting chlamydial infection. These patients should be treated with a combination of penicillin and tetracycline.

Causes of Vaginal Discharge

- *Candida albicans* (curdy discharge)
- *Trichomonas vaginalis*
- Bacterial vaginosis
- *Neisseria gonorrhoeae*
- *Chlamydia trachomatis*
- Herpes simplex
- Non-infective (polyp, cancer, retained products)

Recurrence or Persistent Urethral Discharge

1. Gonococcal discharge. The underlying causes include:
   - Resistance to antibiotics
   - Other causes which has been missed (non-gonococcal urethritis)
   - Re-infection from untreated partner
2. Non-gonococcal urethritis. The underlying causes are as above, but also look for:
   - *Trichomonas vaginalis*
   - *Candida* infection
   - Culture for herpes simplex virus
   - UTI
   - Exclude prostatitis

Gonorrhoea

Gonorrhoea is a sexually transmitted infection affecting the epithelium of the urethra, cervix, rectum and pharynx. The causative agent is *Neisseria gonorrhoeae* that are gram-negative, kidney-shaped intracellular diplococci. Up to 50 per cent of infected women are asymptomatic. Once infected women frequently act as asymptomatic carriers for weeks or months. Homosexual men may also act as carriers in the oropharynx and rectum.

Symptoms and signs

The incubation period is from 2 to 14 days (men) and 7 to 21 days (women). Dysuria, purulent yellowish green urethral or vaginal discharge and urgency of micturition develop. Rectal gonorrhoea is seen in women or homosexual men and presents with perianal discomfort, pain on defecation or rectal intercourse.

Diagnosis

- Gram-stain of genital exudate allows rapid identification of the gonococcus
- Identification of the gonococcus by culture in a medium (such as modified Thayer-Martin medium)
- Tests for *Chlamydia* and syphilis should be obtained at the time of diagnosis and in three months and the patient should be thoroughly examined to exclude other sexually transmitted diseases.

Complications

- Post-non-gonococcal urethritis is due to *Chlamydia trachomatis* infection, which was acquired simultaneously with gonococcus. *Chlamydia* has a longer incubation period and does not respond to penicillins and cefalosporins. Typically, the chlamydial discharge and dysuria are less dramatic and occur 7 to 14 days after penicillin treatment for gonorrhoea.
- Epididymitis (usually unilateral)
- Periurethral abscess
- Prostatitis
- Urethral stricture
- Salpingitis (women)
- Disseminated gonococcal infection
- Arthritis-dermatitis syndrome (a mild febrile illness, migratory polyarthralgia, a few pustular skin lesions on the limbs).
- Pericarditis, endocarditis, meningitis and perihepatitis rarely.
- Gonococcal arthritis (acute onset with fever, pain, and involvement of one or few joints, with synovial fluid showing gonococci).
- Ocular infections occur in the newborn and can be prevented by prophylaxis.

Treatment

- Uncomplicated gonococcal infection: single intramuscular 125 mg dose of ceftriaxone or single oral 500 mg dose of ciprofloxacin (or 400 mg of ofloxacin). First choice of antibiotic depends on local sensitivity profile.
- Patients in whom the above is contraindicated (due to allergy or pregnancy) can be given a single intramuscular 2 g dose of spectinomycin.
- Disseminated gonococcal infection: parenteral ceftriaxone, cefotaxime, ciprofloxacin or ofloxacin for 5 to 7 days
- Other measures:
  - Advise patients to abstain from sexual activity until treatment is completed.
  - Trace the patient's sexual contacts and treat if any evidence of infection.
  - Test of cure is advised to confirm eradication. Because of risk of re-infection, re-test patients in 1 to 2 months.
  - Look for associated sexually transmitted infections such as chlamydial and HIV infections.

Case 88

Multiple Sclerosis

A 42-year-old housewife attended the A and E department with double vision and headache of two days duration. There was no history of nausea or vomiting. Clinically there was no meningeal irritation. Eye movements showed impaired adduction of the left eye and nystagmus of the right eye on right lateral gaze. There was mild dysmetria in both hands. Both plantars were extensor. Six weeks ago, she had numbness of the right arm during which time a CT brain was normal. This resolved completely. An urgent MRI scan was arranged (the result is shown below).

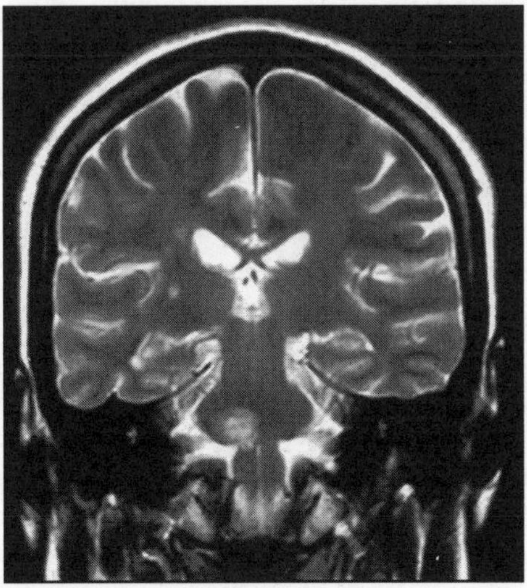

What is the most likely diagnosis?

A. Pontine glioma
B. Amyotrophic lateral sclerosis
C. Multiple sclerosis

D. Wernicke's encephalopathy
E. Lateral medullary syndrome

Answer (C)

DISCUSSION

Multiple Sclerosis

This woman has features of an internuclear ophthalmoplegia (diplopia, impaired adduction of the left eye), cerebellar signs (nystagmus, dysmetria), pyramidal signs (extensor plantar responses) and sensory symptoms (numbness right hand). She has presented to her doctors on two separate occasions and the symptoms were widely distributed in the CNS. Symptoms or signs, which are separated by time and neuroanatomy, suggest the diagnosis of MS.

- MS occurs most commonly in the northern hemisphere, especially between the ages of 20 and 40 years, and women out-number men by 2:1. The disease progresses faster in men and older people.
- In England and Wales, there are 63,000 patients with MS.
- The aetiology is unknown: perivascular inflammation produces plaques of demyelination in the white matter of the spinal cord and brain, which appear as areas of high T2 signal on the MRI scan.
- The constant formation of new demyelinating plaques leads to disease exacerbations: these symptomatic episodes are therefore, separated by time and the associated signs occur in widely different neurological locations. The course of the disease may be relapsing and remitting "RRMS" (i.e. acute episodes that improve), or progressive (i.e. gradual progression without remissions). Progressive disease may occur from the onset (Primary Progressive MS, or "PPMS") or may intervene after many years of the RRMS variety (Secondary Progressive, or "SPMS").
- The Expanded Disability Status Scale (EDSS) is a non-linear scale (0 to 10 in half units) for recording the progression of the disease and is used in research trials: 0 = no neurological disability; 7 = restricted to wheelchair; 8.5 = bed bound; 10 = death.

- The common sites for demyelination are:
  - Optic neuritis (ocular pain, blurred vision or acute loss of vision, colour desaturation especially the loss of red colour perception and swelling of the optic disc).
  - Retrobulbar neuritis (i.e. involvement of the optic nerve before it enters the eye (so there is visual loss without any obvious optic disc oedema).
  - *Devic disease is an acute form of MS presenting as optic neuritis and transverse myelitis.*
  - Spinal cord involvement is particularly common in patients with the progressive form of MS and leads to paraplegia and incontinence.
  - Frontal lobe involvement (severe fatigue, depression, dementia) can occur both early and late in the disease.
  - Brain stem and cerebellum (facial palsy, trigeminal neuralgia, vertigo, nystagmus, ataxia and internuclear ophthalmoplegia). Bilateral facial palsy and trigeminal neuralgia strongly suggest MS.

Diagnostic tests

- CSF Oligoclonal bands: IgG produced by inflammatory cells appear on electrophoresis as oligoclonal bands
- MRI scan
- Evoked potentials: visual evoked potentials

Treatment

- Symptom control: physiotherapy, occupational therapy, speech therapy, muscle relaxants, antidepressants, etc.
- Steroids for acute relapses: IV methylprednisolone 1 gram daily for 3 to 5 days may be better than oral corticosteroids.
- Disease modifying treatment:
  - Beta-interferons: beta-1a interferon (Avonex) and beta-1b interferon (Betaferon) increase the levels of TGF-beta, which has anti-inflammatory properties. Both drugs are given parenterally and cause flu-like symptoms.
  - Glatiramer (Copaxone) resemble myelin proteins and possibly divert lymphocytes away from their inflammatory attack on brain tissue. It is given subcutaneously and produces flushing and chest tightness as side effects.

In RRMS, beta-interferons and glatiramer have been shown to reduce relapse rates by 30 per cent over 2 years. The report from the National Institute of Clinical Excellence (NICE) in January 2002, after reviewing clinical and cost effectiveness, concluded that neither beta-interferon nor glatiramer is recommended for the treatment of MS in the England and Wales.

REFERENCE

1. Beta-interferon and glatiramer acetate for the treatment of multiple sclerosis, technology appraisal no. 32, NICE Jan 2002. (www.nice.org.uk).

Case 89

Guillain-Barré Syndrome

A 44-year-old man complained of progressive weakness of the arms and legs over five days. He could not climb stairs and had been falling at home. The only recent medical illness was flu like symptoms two weeks ago. The temperature was 37.8° Celsius, blood pressure 120/78 mmHg and heart rate 100 bpm. The respiratory rate was 40 per minute and shallow. He was alert with no cranial nerve palsies. There was flaccid weakness of the muscles of the shoulder and pelvis. The tendon reflexes were absent. There was no sensory loss and both plantars were flexor.

What is the most likely diagnosis?

A. Acute polymyositis
B. Myasthenia gravis
C. Guillain-Barré syndrome
D. Transverse myelitis
E. Subacute combined degeneration of the cord

Answer (C)

DISCUSSION

Guillain-Barré Syndrome

Guillain-Barré syndrome (GBS) refers to a group of inflammatory demyelinating polyneuropathies due to immune mediated mechanisms. The overall incidence of GBS is around 1 to 2 cases per 100,000 each year. The average age of onset is 40 years, but the disease occurs in all age groups. In two third of patients there is an antecedent acute respiratory or diarrhoeal illness. Antibodies raised against these invading pathogens are thought to cross react with nerve tissue: a phenomenon called molecular mimicry. Anti-myelin antibodies and complement lock onto and destroy the myelin sheath surrounding peripheral nerves, leading to segmental demyelination, and decreased nerve conduction. Severe cases will progress to axonal degeneration and Wallerian degeneration.

- *Campylobacter jejuni* enteritis is the most common antecedent infection in GBS and may account for one quarter of all cases.
- GBS can also complicate many viral infections, such as influenza, coxsackie, Epstein- Barr, CMV, herpes simplex, HBV and HIV.
- Cases of GBS are rarely precipitated by vaccination to influenza, measles, mumps, rubella and rabies.
- Pregnancy (especially the last trimester) and the puerperium.

Types of GBS

- Acute inflammatory demyelinating poly (radiculo) neuropathy (AIDP). This is the most common type:
  - There is an ascending paralysis with weakness starting in the feet which progresses to affect all 4 limbs, face and oropharyngeal and respiratory muscles.
  - Also common are sensory symptoms such as tingling paraesthesiae (but signs of sensory loss are mild) and low back pain.
  - Autonomic involvement (tachycardia, postural hypotension, hypertension, labile blood pressures, cardiac arrest, cardiac arrhythmias, sweating, urinary retention and constipation).
  - Pathologically the main finding is segmental demyelination, which may be accompanied by some axonal nerve loss.
- Acute motor axonal neuropathy (AMAN)
  - This is a pure motor variety, which presents with weakness only and without any sensory nerve involvement. Antibodies against ganglioside GM1 are often found.
- Acute motor and sensory axonal neuropathy (AMSAN)
  - AMSAN presents with motor and sensory nerve involvement. The pathology of AMAN and AMSAN is predominantly axonal degeneration and Wallerian degeneration, and the myelin sheath is relatively spared, i.e. the opposite of that seen in AIDP. Despite these

differences in pathological findings, the clinical manifestations in AMSAN are similar to AIDP.

- Miller Fisher syndrome.
  - This presents as ataxia, areflexia, and ophthalmoplegia due to demyelination of the III and VI cranial nerves. There is mild limb weakness. The Miller Fisher variant is commoner in children (20% of cases) compared with adults (less than 5% of patients). Antibodies against ganglioside GQ1b are found in this subtype.
- Acute panautonomic neuropathy
  - This is the least common form of GBS. The autonomic manifestations are those described for AIDP.

Diagnostic tests

- Nerve conduction studies (NCS). In Guillain-Barré syndrome, NCS may show the following features of demyelination: reduced conduction velocity (but can be normal in the early stage), conduction block, prolonged latencies, prolonged F waves.
- IgG anti-ganglioside antibodies: anti-GM1 antibodies in motor variant of Guillain-Barré syndrome and anti-GQ1b antibodies in the Miller Fisher syndrome.
- CSF studies. The typical CSF finding in GBS is an elevated protein level without an increase in white cell count. Typically, there are less than 10 white cells per mm^3. However, the CSF may be normal if examined in the first week.
- Stool culture for *Campylobacter jejuni.*

Exclusion of other causes of motor weakness

- Heavy metal poisoning (lead, mercury)
- Poliomyelitis
- Diphtheria
- Porphyria
- Spinal cord compression
- Transverse myelitis
- Botulism
- Organophosphate poisoning
- Hypophosphataemia

Treatment of GBS

These patients require close monitoring and supportive care. They are best managed in a HDU or ITU. Mechanical ventilatory support is needed in about 30 per cent of all GBS patients.

- Consider intubation if the FVC is < 60 per cent of the predicted value, or if the FVC is < 15 ml/kg.
- Thromboembolic disease prophylaxis: heparin
- Plasmapheresis
- IV immunoglobulin (400 mg/kg daily for 5 days).
- Physical therapy
- Note: corticosteroids are considered to be no longer useful in GBS.

Prognosis

Full recovery is seen in about 75 to 85 per cent of patients within 6 to 12 months. Permanent neurological damage occurs in 10 per cent such as hand muscle wasting and weakness, foot drop, sensory ataxia, paraesthesiae and chronic fatigue. The mortality rate is under 5 per cent in centres of excellence and the causes of death are cardiac arrest, pneumonia and pulmonary embolism. Poor prognostic groups are the elderly, pre-existing cardio-respiratory disease, rapidly progressive neurological disease with severely abnormal nerve conduction findings, patients requiring intubation and delays in starting immune therapy with either plasmapheresis or immunoglobulin (both are equally effective). Another 5 per cent will relapse after making a recovery.

Case 90

Miller Fisher Syndrome

An 80-year-old man was given antibiotics for a chest infection by his General Practitioner. Two weeks later, he developed difficulty swallowing and had a choking fit while eating a sandwich. He took to his bed, complained of back pain, bilateral leg pain, numbness in the feet, and became doubly incontinent. He smoked 20 cigarettes a day and drank 20 units of alcohol each week. Past medical history included bilateral hip replacements and osteoarthritis of both knees. On examination, he was confused with slurred speech. Bronchial breathing was present at the base of the right lung. There was bilateral ptosis, ophthalmoplegia, and mild proximal weakness in both legs. All tendon reflexes were absent and the plantar responses were equivocal. He did not co-operate with sensory examination. The bladder was palpable up to the level of the umbilicus. The prostate was smoothly enlarged and the rectum impacted with faeces.

What is the most likely diagnosis?

A. Guillain-Barré syndrome
B. Wernicke's encephalopathy
C. Myasthenia gravis
D. Poliomyelitis
E. Polymyositis
F. Diphtheria
G. Botulism

Answer (A)

DISCUSSION

- The Miller Fisher variant of Guillain-Barré syndrome is the most likely diagnosis (see discussion in case 2).

- Wernicke's encephalopathy should be considered in view of this patient's high alcohol intake and signs of ophthalmoplegia, but dysphagia is not a recognised feature.
- Other causes of muscle weakness accompanied by ptosis and bulbar symptoms include myasthenia gravis, Eaton-Lambert syndrome, poliomyelitis, diphtheria, and botulism.
- Polymyositis does not involve the ocular muscles.
- Sensory symptoms such as numbness do not feature in myasthenia gravis, Eaton-Lambert syndrome, poliomyelitis and botulism.
- Diphtheria is a rarity in the modern vaccine era, but its neurological features and CSF findings are indistinguishable from Guillain-Barré syndrome.

The patient also has signs of consolidation in the right lung and in the context of someone with difficulty swallowing aspiration, pneumonia is likely.

The essential investigations are therefore:

- Chest X-ray
- Blood tests including serum electrolytes, calcium, LFT, PSA
- Arterial blood gases
- Spirometry and measurement of FVC
- Lumbar puncture and CSF analysis
- Nerve conduction studies
- IgG anti-ganglioside antibodies: Anti-GQ1b antibody is described in the Miller Fisher syndrome.

Case 91

Visual Field Defect

A 45-year-old woman suddenly developed visual loss while driving and narrowly missed being involved in an accident. Assessment in the A and E department showed no obvious abnormalities of visual acuity, papillary responses to light and accommodation and optic fundi. She was referred to the local Eye Hospital, where a more detailed examination showed a left homonymous hemianopia.

Where is the likely site of the lesion?

A. Left optic nerve
B. Optic chiasma
C. Right optic tract or right optic radiation
D. Left Macula
E. Edinger-Westphal nucleus

Answer (C)

DISCUSSION

Visual Pathway and Visual Field Defects

The following numbers refer to those in the diagram of the visual pathways and visual field defects.

1. Lesion of the optic nerve: total blindness.
2. Lesion at the optic chiasma: bitemporal hemianopia due to damage to the decussating fibres from the nasal retina in both eyes.
3. Lesion of the optic tract: *incongruous* homonymous hemianopia (*incongruous* means the defects in visual field are not symmetrical and much greater on the side of the lesion).

4. Lesion of the lower part of the optic radiation or Meyer's loop in the temporal lobe (Meyer's loop refers to the fibres of optic radiation that pass forward into the temporal lobe and over the tip of the temporal horn of the lateral ventricle before turning back beneath the ventricle to terminate in the inferior part of the calcarine sulcus of the occipital cortex): homonymous superior quadrinopia.
5. Lesion of the optic radiation in the parietal lobe: homonymous inferior quadrinopia.
6. Lesion of the occipital lobe: highly *congruous* homonymous hemianopia. A *congruous* homonymous hemianopia is one in which the defects in the visual field in each eye are symmetrical in position, shape, size, and degree. Highly *congruous* homonymous hemianopia suggest a lesion in the occipital cortex. The macula is bilaterally represented at the visual cortex: consequently, macular vision spared in a unilateral lesion.

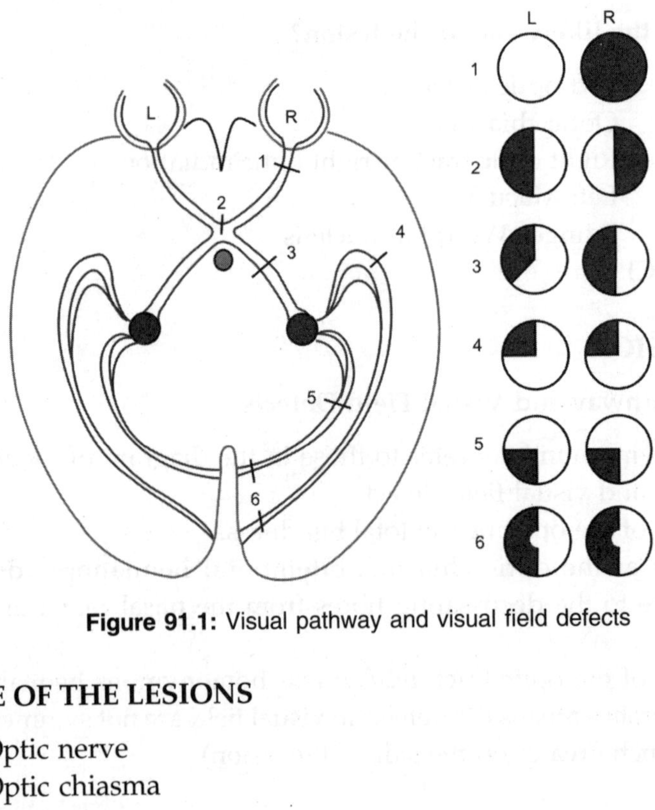

Figure 91.1: Visual pathway and visual field defects

SITE OF THE LESIONS

1. Optic nerve
2. Optic chiasma
3. Optic tract
4. Optic radiation - temporal lobe

5. Optic radiation - parietal lobe
6. Occipital lobe

LINKS TO BOOK ONE

1. Case 42, page 130. Polycythaemia vera
2. Case 72, page 237. Cortical blindness
3. Case 73, page 239. Weber's syndrome
4. Case 88, page 298. Carotid artery dissection
5. Case 91, page 309. Stroke in a young patient

Case 92

Millard-Gubler Syndrome

A 75-year-old man was admitted with sudden onset of headache and diplopia. One hour later he complained of dizziness, started vomiting and developed weakness of the left arm and left leg. When examined in detail he was found to have weakness of the right side of the face, a left hemiplegia, and a left Babinski response.

What is the most likely diagnosis?

A. Weber syndrome
B. Brown-Séquard syndrome
C. Millard-Gubler syndrome
D. Lateral medullary syndrome
E. Basilar artery occlusion

Answer (C)

DISCUSSION

This patient has a right facial palsy of the lower motor neurone type and a 'crossed' left hemiparesis. This is called Millard-Gubler syndrome and the lesion is located in the right side of the pons. It is one of the many brainstem syndromes.

Brainstem Syndromes

The key features of brainstem syndromes are:

- Ipsilateral cranial nerve signs, i.e. located on the same side as the lesion.
- Contralateral or 'crossed' hemiplegia, due to the involvement of the corticospinal tracts destined for the limbs on the opposite side of the body.

- The aetiology of these syndromes is usually a vascular lesion, i.e. occlusion of branches of the vertebral and basilar arteries, or tumour.

LINKS TO BOOK ONE

Case 73, page 239. Weber's syndrome
Case 88, page 298. Carotid artery dissection
Case 91, page 309. Stroke in a young patient

The following table describes some of the eponymous syndromes that present with contralateral or 'crossed' hemiplegia:

Eponym	*Site of lesion*	*Cranial nerve affected*	*Major Neurological Signs*
Parinaud	High Midbrain		Paralysis of upward gaze and accommodation Retraction nystagmus Pupillary areflexia
Weber	Midbrain	III	Ipsilateral oculomotor palsy + contralateral hemiplegia
Benedict	Midbrain	III	Ipsilateral oculomotor palsy + contralateral ataxia and rubral tremor (due to involvement of the superior cerebral peduncle and red nucleus) + contralateral hemiplegia
Millard-Gubler	Pons	VII +/- VI	Ipsilateral facial palsy + contralateral hemiplegia
Foville	Pons	VII	Ipsilateral facial palsy + conjugate lateral gaze palsy (to side of lesion)
Avellis	Medulla	X	Ipsilateral paralysis of palate and vocal cord + contralateral hemianaesthesia (spinothalamic) + contralateral hemiplegia
Jackson	Medulla	X, XI, XII	Ipsilateral paralysis of palate and vocal cord Ipsilateral weakness of sternomastoid and trapezius Ipsilateral weakness of tongue + contralateral hemiplegia
Wallenberg	Medulla + adjacent parts of cerebellum + Spinothalamic tracts	Spinal nucleus of V, IX, X	Ipsilateral facial pain and temp sensory loss Ipsilateral paralysis of palate and vocal cord Ipsilateral ataxia and nystagmus Ipsilateral Horner's syndrome + contralateral spinothalamic sensory loss + contralateral hemiparesis (mild)*

* Contralateral hemiparesis is unusual in lateral medullary syndrome but when present it is mild

Case 93

Myasthenia Gravis

A 29-year-old housewife was referred by her General Practitioner for investigation of excessive tiredness and double vision. She experienced difficulty swallowing and choked on her food and drink. Her symptoms started two weeks ago and were always worse in the evenings. A urinary tract infection was treated one week earlier. She did not smoke and was teetotal. There was no significant past medical history. On examination, she had signs of bilateral partial ptosis, diplopia on lateral gaze and slurred speech. The tendon reflexes were generally depressed, but the plantar responses were flexor. Peripheral sensation was not impaired.

What is the most likely diagnosis?

A. Guillain-Barré syndrome
B. Acute viral polymyositis
C. Myasthenia gravis
D. Acute intermittent porphyria
E. Acute disseminated encephalomyelitis

Answer (C)

DISCUSSION

Myasthenia Gravis

This patient has weakness of the ocular (diplopia) and bulbar muscles (dysphagia). There was no sensory disturbance. The excessive tiredness and double vision in the evenings immediately suggest the muscular fatigability that is typical of myasthenia gravis (MG). Lymphoid hyperplasia in the thymus is found. About 10 per cent of patients with MG will have a thymoma, which is generally benign but can become malignant.

- MG is characterised by muscle weakness and fatigue. Muscle wasting may occur later on. The heart is not affected. The incidence is about two cases in one million. The disease can occur at any age, but the mean age of onset is 30 to 40 years, with a preponderance of females.
- The muscles affected include those of the proximal limb; face (bilateral facial weakness); ocular area (ptosis, diplopia, and squint); and bulbar area (nasal voice or nasal regurgitation due to weak palate, weakness of the jaw after prolonged chewing, pharyngeal weakness and dysphagia).
- The most dangerous situation is involvement of the respiratory muscles leading to acute respiratory failure. Intercurrent illness and many drugs can exacerbate MG including: antibiotics (aminoglycosides, ciprofloxacin, erythromycin, ampicillin); anti-arrhythmics (beta-blockers, verapamil, procainamide, quinidine, magnesium); neuromuscular blockers.
- The myasthenic process may remain confined to the ocular muscles (15% of patients) or become generalised (the remaining 85%).
- MG is an autoimmune disease. IgG antibodies are directed against acetylcholine receptor (AChR) proteins on the postsynaptic membrane, leading to complement mediated destruction of these receptors at the neuromuscular junction. These AChR antibodies cross the placenta and can produce neonatal myasthenia. Other autoimmune diseases can appear in patients with MG, including rheumatoid arthritis, thyrotoxicosis, lupus, scleroderma and red cell aplasia.
- AChR antibodies, which are produced by B-cells, are present in > 90 per cent of patients with idiopathic MG, but may be absent in those with pure ocular MG. They also occur in people with penicillamine induced MG. Anti-striated muscle (Anti-SM) antibody is common in young patients with a thymoma.
- Edrophonium (Tensilon) is an anticholinesterase. A test dose of 2 mg is given IV, followed by another 8 mg IV. Atropine IV 0.6 mg will abolish the bradycardic adverse effect due to edrophonium. A positive test is associated with a marked short lived improvement in muscle strength.
- EMG shows a pattern of decreasing muscle action potential.
- A thymoma may be present on a chest X-ray or CT chest.

- Oral anticholinesterases form the basis of medical treatment: e.g. pyridostigmine 60 mg 4 to 6 hourly. Patients with a poor response to anticholinesterase require corticosteroids often combined with azathioprine. Anti-osteoporosis measures are needed as in any patient on long-term corticosteroids.
- Thymectomy may improve myasthenic symptoms in 40 to 60 per cent of patients without a thymic tumour and 50 per cent of patients obtain remission after 5 years. Thymectomy in those with a tumour is mandatory to exclude malignancy, but may not improve symptoms. The mechanism by which thymectomy improves myasthenia is unclear, but some studies show a fall in acetylcholine receptor antibody levels after the operation.
- Plasma exchange or plasmapheresis is useful for acute episodes of weakness.

Eaton-Lambert Syndrome (ELS) or myasthenic syndrome

- The ELS syndrome is seen in about two per cent of patients with oat cell carcinoma of the lung. This is the most common malignancy linked to ELS. Symptoms of muscular weakness can precede the presentation of the lung malignancy.
- Other associated malignancies are carcinomas of the breast, malignant thymoma, bladder, ovary and gastrointestinal tract.
- The muscle weakness is due to defective release of Acetylcholine (ACh) from the presynaptic part of the neuromuscular junction. The disease has an autoimmune basis and IgG autoantibodies are directed at the voltage-gated calcium channel, which are located presynaptically and are important for ACh release.
- Proximal limb weakness, especially the thigh muscles, is prominent and progressive. Ptosis and dysphagia are due to ocular and bulbar muscle involvement and cause diagnostic confusion with myasthenia gravis (MG). Respiratory muscle function is less severely affected in ELS compared with MG
- Facilitation is a characteristic feature in ELS and describes the improvement in muscle strength with exercise, but this can also occur in the proximal muscles in myasthenia. Tendon reflexes in ELS may be absent on initial examination, but reappear when tested after exercise.

- The most important differential diagnosis is MG: ACh receptor antibody test (positive in MG, but negative in ELS), Tensilon test (markedly positive in MG, but less dramatic in ELS) and EMG (see below) are helpful.
- The EMG in ELS is characteristic: repeated stimulation of the motor nerve produces an increase in muscle response.
- Treatment directed at tumour improves symptoms e.g. chemotherapy or radiotherapy for oat cell lung tumour.
- Plasmapheresis and immunotherapy (prednisolone and azathioprine) improve the muscle weakness.
- The response to guanidine (which improves ACh release) and anticholinesterase (e.g. pyridostigmine) is variable.
- Aminoglycosides and calcium channel blocker may worsen symptoms in patients with ELS. Symptoms also worsen in hot weather.
- The main cause of death in ELS is the underlying malignancy.

LINKS TO BOOK ONE

1. Case 63, page 199. Hypogammaglobulinaemia (Good's syndrome = thymoma and immunodeficiency).

Case 94

Idiopathic Intracranial Hypertension

An 18-year-old university student presented with a 3 weeks history of frontal headache. There was no vomiting or visual disturbance. She was taking the oral contraceptive pill, but no other medications. There was no significant past medical problems. On examination, she was overweight, the blood pressure was 122/78 mmHg, and fundoscopy showed pink optic discs. An urgent CT brain was normal.

What is the most likely diagnosis?

A. Benign intracranial hypertension
B. Migraine
C. Tension headache
D. Bilateral optic neuritis
E. Posterior communicating aneurysm

Answer (A)

DISCUSSION

Benign Intracranial Hypertension

Benign intracranial hypertension is also called idiopathic intracranial hypertension (IIH) or "pseudotumour cerebri". The annual incidence of IIH is 1 per 100,000 of the population, with a female to male ratio of 8 to 1, and affected individuals tend to be obese young women. The chronically elevated intracranial pressure is due to increased resistance in the absorption of the CSF at the level of the arachnoid villi granulations. Although the symptoms in these patients may initially suggest a brain tumour, the CT and MRI brain scans are reassuringly normal and this gave rise to the old description of "pseudotumour cerebri". MRI and MR venography will also rule out another important cause of raised intracranial hypertension, namely cerebral sinus thrombosis, which may be missed by CT.

The essential points in the diagnosis of IHH are:

- Symptoms and signs of raised intracranial pressure (see below)
- Normal neuro-imaging (CT or MRI)
- Raised CSF pressure (> 25 cm of water in the lateral position). Note: the *normal* CSF opening pressure is about 50 cm of water if the lumbar puncture is performed in a sitting position.
- Normal CSF fluid analysis

Chronically elevated intracranial pressure in IHH produces the following symptoms and signs:

- Headache
- Tinnitus which is exacerbated by changes in posture
- Transient visual obscurations (momentary dimming of vision induced by changes in posture, e.g. stooping, or Valsalva) indicate critical optic nerve ischaemia
- Loss of colour vision
- Visual acuity is initially normal, but there is progressive loss of peripheral vision (starting in the infra-nasal region)
- Double vision due to unilateral or bilateral VI nerve palsy (this is a false localising sign in intracranial hypertension)
- Papilloedema (swollen optic discs): enlarged blind spot is an early sign. Other causes of swollen optic discs are malignant hypertension, optic neuritis, and drusen of the optic nerves.
- Optic neuropathy, i.e. optic atrophy with blindness, is the final result of chronic papilloedema

Idiopathic intracranial hypertension is associated with the following:

- Obesity, including recent weight gain
- Endocrine disease: hypothyroidism, hypoparathyroidism, Addison's disease, Cushing's disease
- Pregnancy
- Medications: oral contraceptive pill, corticosteroid treatment (administered orally or topically), corticosteroid withdrawal (an unexplained paradox), tetracycline, vitamin A, isotretinoin, recombinant human growth hormone, nitrofurantoin, trimethoprim-sulfamethoxazole, amiodarone, lithium
- Chronic respiratory failure, renal failure
- Anticardiolipin antibodies and lupus anticoagulant may be

found
- Systemic lupus erythematosus (SLE)

Treatment

- Treat the underlying cause. Some cases remit spontaneously or improve with medication, but the possibility of recurrence will necessitate long-term follow up.
- Encourage weight loss.
- Lumbar puncture is done after exclusion of an intracranial mass lesion. The opening CSF pressure is measured and the fluid analysed.
- Acetazolamide 250 mg qds orally. Frusemide is an alternative for those who are intolerant to acetazolamide, but is less effective in lowering intracranial pressure.
- Corticosteroids lower CSF pressure perhaps by facilitating outflow at arachnoid granulations and can be combined with acetazolamide. Patients with progressive loss of visual field can be given high dose prednisolone (60 mg od initially and tapered according to response) and referred for CSF shunting or optic nerve sheath fenestration.
- Lumboperitoneal, ventriculoperitoneal, or ventriculoatrial shunts.
- Optic nerve sheath fenestration: slits are made in the dura surrounding the optic nerve immediately behind the globe, which allow the CSF to escape into the orbital fat.

Case 95

Tuberculous Meningitis

A 17-year-old Indian student was visiting his uncle's family in England. He had been complaining of headaches over the last two days and became drowsy. No past medical history was available. On examination, he was apyrexial and sleepy, but easily rousable. Neck movements were uncomfortable. There was no skin rash, lymphadenopathy or hepatomegaly.

Hb	14.2 g/dl	
WBC	$4 \times 10^9/l$	
Platelets	$241 \times 10^9/l$	
Na	148 mmol/l	
K	4.8 mmol/l	
Urea	8.2 mmol/l	
Creatinine	111 μmol/l	
Glucose	6.0 mmol/l	
CXR	normal	
Urine	trace protein	
Blood film for malaria	negative	
Blood cultures	awaited	
CSF	cells	$64/mm^3$
	protein	0.8 g/l
	glucose	1.2 mmol/l
	gram stain	no bacteria, culture awaited

What is the most likely cause?

A. Herpes simplex encephalitis
B. Mumps encephalitis
C. Poliomyelitis

D. Tuberculous meningitis
E. Acute HIV infection

Answer (D)

DISCUSSION

The CSF showed a pleocytosis, low sugar content and elevated protein concentration, which are suggestive of either bacterial or tuberculous infection. A low CSF glucose may also occur in malignant infiltration of the meninges.

Tuberculous Meningitis

Tuberculous meningitis (TBM) is due to the haematogenous spread of mycobacteria from the lungs to the CNS. Caseous lesions are found in the brain parenchyma (which produce tuberculoma or abscess) and on the meninges (which rupture into the subarachnoid space to produce meningitis). Cranial nerve dysfunction, obstruction to the flow of CSF, and vasculitic infarction are the inevitable consequence of this meningeal inflammatory reaction.

Symptoms and signs

- Confusion and drowsiness of gradual onset
- Headache and vomiting
- Neck stiffness may be mild or absent
- Seizures
- Papilloedema
- Retinal choroid tubercles
- Vasculitic infarction can produce: hemiplegia, monoplegia, aphasia
- Cranial nerve palsies: III, IV, VII

Diagnosis

- Consider TB in susceptible groups, e.g. diabetics, patients on long-term corticosteriod therapy, alcoholics, vagrants, HIV, malnutrition, socio-economic deprivation, underlying malignancy, ethnic individuals from countries where TB is commoner.
- Differentiation from other types of subacute meningitis may be difficult, including viral, fungal, brucella, syphilis and Lyme's disease.

- Chest X-ray: hilar lymphadenopathy, effusions, infiltration, cavities, miliary opacities.
- Lumbar puncture: CSF mycobacterial culture currently takes 4 weeks. Mycobacterial DNA can be identified using polymerase chain reaction in a couple of days.
- CT and MRI: hydrocephalus, tuberculoma, infarcts, and oedema.

Chemotherapy

- Isoniazid (INH), rifampicin (RIF), pyrazinamide (PZA), and streptomycin will all cross the blood brain barrier. Ethambutol is less effective. A common regime is INH + RIF + PZA for 6 to 9 months
- The role of corticosteroids is unclear.

LINKS TO BOOK ONE

1. Case 25, page 72. Lymphocytic meningitis.

Case 96

Temporal Lobe Epilepsy

A 56-year-old anatomy lecturer whose professional conduct had previously been impeccable was seen undressing in the college corridor. He was quietly taken to the neurology department. He complained there was a strong smell of rotting fish in the consulting room. On arrival, he was lethargic but rousable. After an hour, he became alert but had gaps in memory about his normal duties for the day.

What is the likely diagnosis?

A. Korsakoff psychosis
B. Petit mal epilepsy
C. Acute delirium
D. Temporal lobe epilepsy
E. Jacksonian epilepsy

Answer (D)

DISCUSSION

This patient has temporal lobe epilepsy presenting as complex partial seizure. The typical features are the olfactory aura of rotting fish and undressing form of automatism. The patient has no recollection of events as both temporal lobes are affected in complex partial seizure.

Epilepsy and a Simplified Classification

Epilepsy is a tendency to have *recurrent* and *unprovoked* seizures. One single seizure is insufficient for the diagnosis of epilepsy. Provoked seizures i.e. those precipitated by fever in children, alcohol, drug abuse, acute stroke, hypoglycaemia and other metabolic conditions, and occurring within seconds of a head injury, are also not included under the term epilepsy.

Epilepsy can be simply divided into the two broad main types:

I Partial seizures, which originate from localised areas of the cortex:
- Simple partial
- Complex partial
- Secondary generalised

II Generalised seizures which originate from both hemispheres:
- Absence seizures ('petit mal')
- Myoclonic seizures
- Clonic seizures
- Tonic seizures
- Tonic-clonic seizures ('grand mal')
- Atonic seizures

Temporal lobe epilepsy

Temporal lobe epilepsy is an example of a partial seizure. Partial seizures are associated with focal manifestations or "auras":
- Sensory: all special senses are affected: flashing lights, distortion of size and shape of objects, vertigo, unpleasant odours or tastes, musical tunes
- Psychic: déjà vu, jamais vu, fear, anxiety, anger, pleasure, recall of old memory fragments, depersonalisation (feelings of detachment), derealisation (environment appear unreal)
- Autonomic: racing heart beat, hypertension, mydriasis, piloerection, nausea, epigastric rising sensation
- Automatisms are involuntary but co-ordinated motor activity and occur in complex partial seizures, e.g. lip smacking, chewing, walking, cycling, dancing, undressing, sexual acts

Cause of Temporal Lobe Epilepsy

- Encephalitis
- Meningitis
- Trauma
- Arteriovenous malformation
- Glioma

- Hippocampal sclerosis is suggested by MRI evidence for hippocampal atrophy. It is bilateral in 15 per cent of patients. A relationship may exist between febrile seizures in childhood, hippocampal sclerosis and temporal lobe epilepsy in later adult life.

Treatment

- Anti-epileptic medication: carbamazepine, valproate, phenytoin, lamotrigine, topiramate. About 40 per cent of patients remain poorly controlled despite 2 or 3 concomitant drugs.
- Vagus nerve stimulation for intractable partial epilepsy may reduce seizure frequency by 25 per cent. It is administered by a battery operated stimulator that has been subcutaneously implanted in the neck. The mechanism of action is not known.
- Temporal lobectomy for patients with intractable TLE. The best results from surgery are seen in patients in whom seizure origin has been confirmed (i.e. MRI showing unilateral hippocampal atrophy and concordant EEG). About 80 to 90 per cent of these patients will be free of seizures after surgery.

LINKS TO BOOK ONE

1. Case 82, page 277. Loss of consciousness and driving.

Case 97

Cysticercosis

A 58-year-old Indian man presented with recurrent epileptic fits in the past two months. They occurred once every two weeks, but he had been reluctant to seek medical help due to the fear of losing his driving licence. This man and his family had immigrated to the UK 10 years ago. His three sons helped him run a successful Indian take away restaurant. He smoked 20 a day, but did not consume alcohol. Clinical examination was unremarkable. In the clinic he was commenced on sodium valproate CR 200 mg bd and further investigations including a CT scan was arranged as an out-patient. Two weeks after his clinic visit, he presented to the A and E department with headache, photophobia and vomiting. An urgent CT brain revealed a few scattered calcified foci of variable sizes in the subcortical area. The ventricles were not dilated. A lumbar puncture showed the following results: white cell count of $78/mm^3$ (50% lymphocytes, 20% neutrophils and 30% eosinophils) and protein concentration of 0.84 g/l. The medical registrar requested X-rays of the lower limbs and these showed areas of calcification in the calf.

What is the most likely cause of the meningitis?

A. *Echinococcus granulosus*
B. Cysticercosis
C. Congenital toxoplasmosis
D. Pseudohypoparathyroidism
E. *Echinococcus* multilocularis

Answer (B)

DISCUSSION

Cysticercosis

Cysticercosis is due to disseminated spread of the larval form of the pork tapeworm, *Taenia Solium,* which is contained in uncooked meat. Once these larval cysts (or cysticerci) are ingested, they can spread to any tissue in the body including the skin (subcutaneous cysts), skeletal muscle (asymptomatic), heart (conduction defects), eyes (vitreous and subretinal cysts) and brain (see below). The tissue inflammatory response to cysticerci is variable, as the parasite seems able to evade host immunity.

Diagnostic tests

- Serology: enzyme-linked immunosorbent assays (ELISA)
- Stool examination for ova and parasites
- Blood and CSF eosinophilia is uncommon
- Imaging: CT or MRI. Cysts with surrounding oedema suggest inflammatory response. MRI may show a nodule within these cysts, which represents the larval scolex. Calcified areas are inactive.
- Biopsy of subcutaneous nodule will be diagnostic

Manifestation of CNS cysticercosis (Neurocysticercosis)

- Headache
- Seizures
- Obstructive hydrocephalus due to cysts in the subarachnoid and ventricles
- Vasculitic infarction

Treatment

- Antihelminthic drug: Albendazole (Albenza) in an oral dose of 15 mg/kg/day (divided bd) for 2 weeks. It kills the parasitic larvae by depleting their ATP energy stores.
- Concomitant administration of corticosteroids is often recommended as the dying parasitic cysts can invoke an inflammatory response
- Long-term anticonvulsants therapy in patients with persistent CNS calcifications.

Case 98

Thrombosis of Posterior Inferior Cerebellar Artery

A 58-year-old engineer presented to A and E department with two weeks of sudden onset dizziness, double vision, headache, vomiting and numbness on the left side of the face. He smoked and was hypertensive for the last three years. His current medications were aspirin 75 mg od, bendroflumethiazide 2.5 mg od and perindopril 2 mg od. He consumed about two pints of beer at weekends. His heart rate was regular at 100 bpm with a blood pressure 170/70 mmHg. The left eye showed a small pupil with partial ptosis. There was nystagmus on looking to left and the patient could not swallow water. Pinprick sensation was reduced on the left side of the face, right arm and leg. There was no hemiplegia. An urgent CT scan did not reveal any space occupying lesion or intracranial haemorrhage.

What is the most likely diagnosis?

A. Total basilar artery occlusion
B. Embolisation to anterior cerebral artery
C. Thrombosis of posterior inferior cerebellar artery
D. Infarction in the posterior cerebral artery
E. Aneurismal rupture of posterior communicating artery

Answer (C)

DISCUSSION

Posterior inferior cerebellar artery thrombosis produces the Wallenburg's syndrome. In this syndrome, the parts of the medulla and adjacent parts of the cerebellum are affected. In addition, the spinothalamic tracts, spinal nuclei of V, IX, X are also affected.

Wallenburg's syndrome has the following elements:

- Ipsilateral facial pain and temp sensory loss
- Ipsilateral paralysis of palate and vocal cord
- Ipsilateral ataxia and nystagmus
- Ipsilateral Horner's syndrome
- Contralateral spinothalamic sensory loss
- Contralateral hemiparesis (mild); this is uncommon.

Horner's syndrome

This has the following features:

- Unilateral papillary constriction
- Partial ptosis
- Enophthalmos
- Anhidrosis (loss of sweating) on the same side of the face

There are numerous causes for Horner's syndrome and it is useful to remember some of the causes mentioned below:

- Cervical sympathectomy
- Cervical rib
- Carotid artery occlusion or dissection (the sympathetic fibres run in the carotid sheath)
- Apical bronchial carcinoma (Pancoast's tumour)
- Malignant infiltration of the brachial plexus
- Massive cerebral infarction
- Lateral medullary syndrome
- Pontine glioma

LINKS TO BOOK ONE

1. Case 73, page 239. Weber's syndrome.
2. Case 88, page 298. Carotid artery dissection.
3. Case 91, page 309. Stroke in a young patient.

Case 99

Migrainous Neuralgia

A previously healthy 44-year-old bank manager was awakened from sleep with severe right eye pain. He has had similar attacks in the last one year, which usually responded to self-medication. He took a couple of paracetamol tablets, but obtained no relief. The pain became much worse and he vomited once. He was a non-smoker and consumed alcohol occasionally. In the A and E department, he was in severe pain with a congested right eye. There was a right partial ptosis, but the eye movements were normal. There was no papilloedema. An urgent assessment at the ophthalmology department excluded acute glaucoma. The sensation over the face was normal. The FBC was normal with a CRP < 10. The CT brain scan was unremarkable.

What is the most likely diagnosis?

A. Giant cell arteritis
B. Facial hemispasm
C. Migrainous neuralgia
D. Trigeminal neuralgia
E. Acute arthritis of the temporomandibular joint

Answer (C)

DISCUSSION

Diagnostic Pit-falls in Acute Severe Headache

Headache is a common symptom: it account for one per cent of visits to General Practitioners and 30 per cent of neurology clinic referrals. One in eight people presenting with sudden severe headache as the only symptom will harbour a subarachnoid haemorrhage – the other seven will have innocuous conditions (Linn el al, Lancet 1994). In this patient the classic symptoms and signs suggested the diagnosis of migrainous neuralgia (also called 'cluster headaches'). A history of previous similar attacks and the absence of pointers to more serious conditions were also reassuring. However, the assessment of patients with sudden onset severe headache is bedevilled by many pitfalls. For example, neck stiffness in SAH may take at least 6 hours to develop and the CT brain scan may not show extravasated blood in two per cent of patients with genuine aneurismal rupture in the previous 12 hours (and in 50% after one week). (Van Gijn, Lancet 1997).

Migrainous Neuralgia

Migrainous neuralgia or cluster headache affects middle-aged men. It is characterised by episodes of severe unilateral periorbital pain (duration 15 -180 minutes), which are accompanied by autonomic phenomena, including nasal congestion, rhinorrhoea, lacrimation, eye redness and Horner's syndrome (ptosis). The term cluster headache describes the pattern: headache occurring daily for several days, which disappear for a variable period, before re-appearing.

Treatment

- Simple analgesia and sumitriptan (6mg s/c) for acute attacks
- Prophylaxis: ergotamine, propranolol and amitriptyline

Other types of short-lived unilateral headache with details of their treatment are:

- Short-lived unilateral headache lasting only for seconds with autonomic features is called SUNCT (= short-lasting, unilateral neuralgiform headache with conjunctival injection and tearing) and may respond to lamotrigine.
- Hemicrania continua and chronic paroxysmal hemicrania respond to indomethacin.

REFERENCES

1. Linn FHH et al. Prospective study of sentinel headache in aneurismal subarachnoid haemorrhage. Lancet 1994;344: 590-93.
2. Van Gijn. Slip-ups in diagnosis of subarachnoid haemorrhage. Lancet 1997; 349: 1492.
3. Goadsby PL and Lipton RB. A review of paroxysmal hemicranias, SUNCT syndrome and other short-lasting headaches with autonomic features, including new cases. Brain 1997; 120: 193-209.

LINKS TO BOOK ONE

1. Case 75, page 246. Subarachnoid haemorrhage.

Case 100

Can He Drive?

An 18-year-old law student has had four seizures in the last three months, two of which were witnessed by paramedics. The biochemical screen and CT brain scan were normal.

Which of the following options would you advise him with regards to driving?

A. He should refrain from driving for 12 months
B. He should not a drive a car, but can drive a motorcycle
C. He can drive if free from seizures for one year while on anticonvulsants
D. One seizure in the next year will not bar him from driving
E. Extra insurance cover will allow him to drive for the next two years

Answer (C)

DISCUSSION

Epilepsy and Driving

Driving is a valuable skill and loss of a driving licence is a serious blow to a person's lifestyle and occupation. In the UK, medical fitness to drive is governed by legislation. Details of medical conditions that affect driving safety are available from the Drivers and Vehicle Licensing Agency (DVLA). An 'At a Glance' booklet is available to all doctors and can be downloaded from the DVLA website (www.dvla.gov.uk). Epileptic attacks are the most common medical cause of collapse at the steering wheel.

The legal position in the UK

- A driving licence is issued and deemed valid until the age of 70 years unless it is revoked by a prescribed medical condition.
- After the age of 70 years, a driving licence is renewed every 3 years.
- The licence holder has a legal obligation to inform the DVLA of any medical condition, which may affect safe driving.
- Doctors must remind patients of their legal obligation to inform the DVLA and document this advice in the patient's record.
- If a patient refuses to accept your medical advice or diagnosis, you should obtain a second medical opinion. You should advise the patient not to drive until the second opinion has been obtained.
- Doctors have a legal obligation to protect the general public and this comes before his duty to protect patient confidentiality. If the patient is acting contrary to medical advice and still driving, you should notify the DVLA and write to the patient that you have done so.
- Group 1 driving licence entitlement refers to Class A (motor cycles) and B (motor cars).
- Group 2 driving licence entitlement refers to Class C (lorries) and D (buses).

Motor Vehicle Classification

In the UK motor vehicles are classified as follows:

• Motor cycles and scooters	Class A
• Motor cars up to 3.5 tonnes carrying 8 or less passengers	Class B
• Lorries and goods vehicles	Class C
- lorries of 3.5 to 7.5 tonnes	Class C1
• Passenger carrying vehicles	Class D
- minibus carrying 16 or less passengers	Class D1
• Mopeds	Class P

Epilepsy and Driving

A patient can reapply for a licence to drive Class A, B, or P vehicles, if:

- Completely free from all seizures for one year
  or seizures have occurred only during sleep for at least 3 years
- As from 1 Jan 1997 licence holders for motor cars (Class B) can also drive a minibus carrying 16 or less passengers (Class D1)

A patient can reapply for a licence to drive Class C or D vehicles, if:

- Holds a full car licence
- Completely free of seizures for 10 years
- Have not had to take anticonvulsant medication during this period and
- Passed a medical review by the DVLA

Taxi driving

- These regulations are generally similar to Class C and D vehicles
- These driving licenses are granted by the local council

Withdrawal of anti-consultant medication

- Compared with those who stayed on treatment, stopping anti-epileptic medication for one year was associated with a 40 per cent increase in risk of seizures
- Patients should be informed of the increased risk of seizure, the consequences of an increased likelihood of road traffic accidents and loss of licence, when coming off anti-epileptic treatment

First Epileptic Seizure or Solitary Fit

- Patient should stop driving
- Patient should notify DVLA
- Normally barred from driving for 1 year
- Needs to be free from all fits for 1 year and must pass a medical review before Group 1 licence is granted
- Needs to be free of all fits for 10 years and off all anticonvulsants during this period before Group 2 licence is granted

Seizures provoked by alcohol and illicit drug misuse

- These cases are considered individually by the DVLA

LINKS TO BOOK ONE

1. Case 82, page 277. Loss of consciousness and driving.

Case 101

Normal Pressure Hydrocephalus

An 82-year-old man presented with intermittent confusion, recurrent falls, difficulty passing urine and incontinence. A CT brain scan was performed.

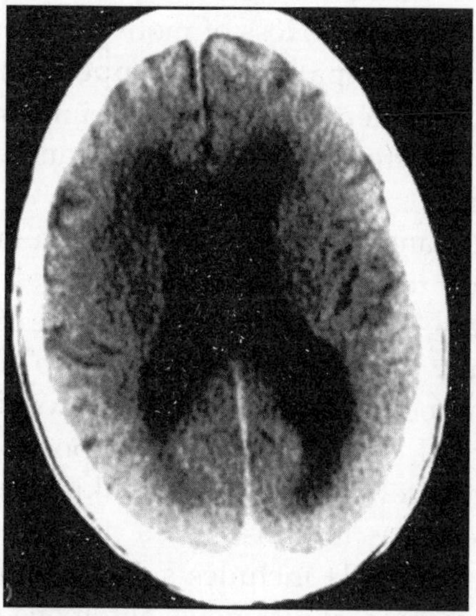

What is the diagnosis?

A. Benign intracranial hypertension
B. Chronic subdural haematoma
C. Normal pressure hydrocephalus
D. Intraventricular bleeding
E. Right frontal lobe glioma multiforme

Answer (C)

DISCUSSION

Normal Pressure Hydrocephalus

Normal pressure hydrocephalus (NPH) is a form of chronic communicating hydrocephalus in adults. The diagnosis of NPH is suggested by the classical triad of:

- dementia
- gait apraxia
- urinary incontinence

By definition, the CSF pressure is normal, but intermittently elevated pressures can be demonstrated at night, leading to damage to the white matter. Headache and papilloedema are not featured in this condition.

The dementia is of the subcortical type with slowing of mental processing, lack of initiative, loss of motivation, hypersomnia, and abulia. Therefore, the patient can appear rather apathetic, emotionally flat, and depressed. Memory impairment is initially mild. The cortical functions such as language and visuospatial skills are usually intact.

The gait disturbance can be described as an inability to lift the legs, as they appear to be stuck to the floor and resemble that seen in Parkinson's disease. This could be due to damage of the basal ganglia from intermittently raised CSF pressures. Drop attacks and loss of consciousness can occur. There is no motor weakness; the tendon reflexes are normal, and the Babinski response absent. Signs of spasticity, hyper-reflexia and Babinski responses indicate concomitant cerebrovascular disease.

The aetiology of NPH includes subarachnoid haemorrhage, trauma, chronic meningeal infections, but in one third, no cause is apparent. The diagnosis is suggested by the following investigations:

- Isotope cisternography. In NPH, radioisotope injected into the lumbar subarachnoid space is abnormally retained in the ventricles for prolonged periods and does not pass normally over the cerebral hemispheres.
- MRI and CT brain scans. Cortical atrophy is absent or less severe than expected for the age of the patient, but the third, fourth and lateral ventricles are enlarged. MRI may also show periventricular transudation of CSF into the brain parenchyma.

- CSF tap test. Patients who show improvement in symptoms following the removal of 30 ml of CSF by lumbar puncture may have a better response to ventriculoperitoneal shunting. Some advocate serial lumbar punctures to effect CSF removal.

In practice, NPH can be difficult to distinguish from other causes of cerebral atrophy and ventricular dilatation and none of the above tests can reliably predict a satisfactory response to ventriculoperitoneal shunting. However, patients with extensive cerebrovascular disease and diffuse atrophy respond poorly to shunting. Postoperative complications such as infection and haemorrhage may occur in 30 per cent of patients who are operated upon.

LINKS TO BOOK ONE

1. Case 22, page 60. Lewy Body Dementia.
2. Case 66, page 213. Acute confusional state.
3. Case 81, page 270. Neuroleptic malignant syndrome.

Case 102

Right Posterior Cerebral Artery

A 32-year-old lady from the Middle-East presented to A and E with sudden onset vertigo, vomiting and collapse. She was known to have mitral valve disease and has had a closed mitral valvotomy 10 years ago. However, she has been left with mild mitral regurgitation and atrial fibrillation. She was on digoxin 250 mcg od and warfarin 4 mg od. Examination in the A and E department showed a left homonymous hemianopia.

Which artery is affected by embolisation?

A. Left vertebral artery
B. Right posterior cerebral artery
C. Left posterior cerebral artery
D. Right posterior inferior cerebellar artery
E. Basilar artery

Answer (B)

DISCUSSION

Lesions of the occipital lobe may produce one or more of the following presentations:

- Visual hallucinations
- Infarction of one occipital pole causes a small congruous (symmetrical) scotoma or congruous homonymous hemianopia (the macular region is spared as it is supplied by the middle cerebral artery)
- Bilateral widespread occipital lobe damage (infarction, haemorrhage, trauma or tumour) results in cortical blindness.

LINKS TO BOOK ONE

1. Case 73, page 239. Weber's syndrome.
2. Case 88, page 298. Carotid artery dissection.
3. Case 91, page 309. Stroke in a young patient.

Case 103

Sleep Apnoea

A 45-year-old lorry driver was admitted to the CCU with an acute myocardial infarction. He did not smoke and took alcohol only occasionally. There were no other cardiovascular risk factors except that he was markedly obese. He received thrombolysis with t-PA followed by heparin infusion for 24 hours. There were no complications. He did not co-operate with his rehabilitation and preferred to spend all day asleep on his bed. He woke up only for meal times, promptly went back to sleep afterwards, and was very bad tempered when disturbed by the nursing staff. At night he slept poorly, snored loudly and kept the other patients awake.

What is the most likely explanation?

A. Narcolepsy
B. Cataplexy
C. Petit mal epilepsy
D. Obstructive sleep apnoea
E. Hepatic encephalopathy

Answer (D)

DISCUSSION

This patient has obstructive sleep apnoea. Narcolepsy describes attacks of irresistible sleep during inappropriate circumstances, mainly after meals or during driving, and may not have an obvious cause. Narcolepsy can be associated with cataplexy, which is a sudden loss of muscle tone leading to fall without loss of consciousness. Both narcolepsy and cataplexy may be associated with:

- Hypnogogic hallucinations which occur while falling asleep
- Hypnopompic hallucinations which occur on waking
- Sleep paralysis which is a frightening inability to move whilst drowsy

Obstructive Sleep Apnoea

Obstructive sleep apnoea (OSA) is defined as sleep induced upper airway obstruction, which leads to symptomatic sleep disturbance and daytime drowsiness. The basic problem is a failure to maintain pharyngeal dilator muscle tone during sleep. The condition is more common in Blacks and Orientals.

Causes of OSA

The following conditions contribute to the narrowing of the upper airways and increase the susceptibility to OSA:

- Obesity: deposition of fat in the neck leads to narrowing of the oropharynx, especially in the space behind the tongue. A neck circumference of 17 inches in men (or 16 inches in women) is a good predictor of OSA.
- Micrognathia: crowded dentition is a useful clue to poor mandibular development.
- Nasal obstruction
- Large tonsils
- Alcohol: reduces muscle tone further
- Smoking
- Acromegaly
- Hypothyroidism
- Neuromuscular disease: stroke, motor neurone disease and muscular dystrophies.

Symptoms of OSA

- Daytime drowsiness leads to poor work performance. Drowsiness behind the steering wheel is responsible for the increased risk of road traffic accidents.
- Loud snoring, choking episodes during sleep and apnoea (noticed by partner).
- Poor quality sleep: sleep is restless, because apnoea is followed by arousal, and there is nocturia due to increased urine production.

- Morning headaches
- Impaired concentration
- Changes in personality and irritability.
- Diminished libido

Severity of OSA

- Apnoea is a 10 second pause in breathing.
- Hypopnoea is a 10 second event during which there is continued breathing but ventilation is reduced by at least 50% from the previous baseline during sleep.
- Apnoea/hypopnoea index (AHI) = the frequency of apnoeas and hypopnoeas hourly.
- Mild OSA = AHI 5-14 per hour
- Moderate OSA = AHI 15-30 per hour
- Severe OSA = AHI > 30 per hour

Investigations

- The severity of sleepiness and its impact on everyday activities can be evaluated using the Epworth Sleepiness Scale. A score of 10 or more indicates possible excessive daytime sleepiness or sleep disorder.
- Sleep study (polysomnography): pulse oximetry, video to record body movements, and microphone to record snoring intensity.
- Hypertension. Marked rises in blood pressure occur during arousals, and the possible long term consequences such as increased risk of stroke or MI require clarification. Daytime hypertension is improved by CPAP (see below).

Treatment

- Encourage patients to lose weight, stop smoking, and avoid alcohol.
- Tonsillectomy if tonsils are greatly enlarged.
- Alleviate nasal obstruction.
- Mandibular advancement device: a mechanical aid to hold the mandible forwards during sleep.
- Nasal continuous positive airway pressure (CPAP).

Continuous positive airway pressure (CPAP)

Pressurised air is given via a small mask worn over the nose. The pressure required to keep the oropharynx patent is 5 to 15 cm of water. The CPAP improves daytime alertness, driving performance and blood pressure.

REFERENCE

1. Management of obstructive sleep apnoea/hypopnoea syndrome in adults. British Thoracic Society and Scottish Intercollegiate Guidelines Network. June 2003 (www.sign.ac.uk).

Epworth Sleepiness Scale
(Johns MW. Sleep 1991;14:540-545)

	Situation	*Chance of Dozing*			
*	Sitting and reading	0	1	2	3
*	Watching TV	0	1	2	3
*	Sitting inactive in a public place e.g. a theatre or meeting	0	1	2	3
*	As a passenger in a car for an hour without a break	0	1	2	3
*	Lying down to rest in the afternoon	0	1	2	3
*	Sitting and talking to someone	0	1	2	3
*	Sitting quietly after lunch (when you've had no alcohol)	0	1	2	3
*	In a car while stopped in traffic	0	1	2	3
		Total score =			

0 = would never doze
1 = slight chance of dozing
2 = moderate chance of dozing
3 = high chance of dozing
ESS total score ≥ 10 indicates possible excessive daytime sleepiness or sleep disorder

Case 104

Arterial Blood Gases (Laboratory Error)

This arterial blood gas result belonged to a lady who was admitted with dyspnoea. The test was taken while breathing room air.

pH	7.54
PaO_2	12.8 kPa
$PaCO_2$	7.5 kPa
HCO_3	14 mmol/l

Which of the following answers is the most likely explanation?

A. Metabolic alkalosis
B. Respiratory acidosis with compensation
C. Respiratory alkalosis
D. Laboratory error
E. Lactic acidosis

Answer (D)

DISCUSSION

All laboratory results should be interpreted in the context of the patient's clinical presentation. In this patient there is apparently an alkalosis (pH = 7.54), a high CO_2, and low HCO_3 – this combination is implausible. See the tips for arterial blood gas interpretation in other examples in this book.

Some common causes for faulty laboratory results are listed below:

- Mis-labeling of samples with serious consequences, including incompatible blood transfusions.
- High serum potassium due to haemolysed blood sample.

- High serum potassium due to "topping up" of an inadequate serum specimen from a full blood count bottle, which contains potassium EDTA as anticoagulant.
- Blood sampling from an IV cannula connected to an infusion.
- Plasma calcium may be falsely high if the blood sample was obtained using an occluding cuff on the arm, as this leads to an increase in local plasma protein concentration.
- Pseudohyponatraemia due to hyperlipidaemia or paraproteinemia.

Case 105

Exercise Induced Asthma

A 15-year-old student was referred to the out-patient clinic for investigation of a dry cough, which had been present for three months. The cough was induced by exertion, especially playing cricket. He was a non-smoker. There was no history of fever, weight loss, or other respiratory symptoms. His elder sister has hay fever. There was no family history of asthma or tuberculosis. On examination, the chest was clear. The chest X-ray, basic blood tests and ECG were normal. Lung function tests showed normal spirometry and lung volumes.

The most likely diagnosis is:

A. Exercise induced asthma
B. Hay fever
C. Pulmonary tuberculosis
D. Congenital heart disease
E. Extrinsic allergic alveolitis

Answer (A)

DISCUSSION

Asthma

Asthma affects 6 per cent of the population. It is an inflammatory condition of the airways with increased bronchial reactivity and airflow obstruction that is reversible spontaneously or with treatment. There is often a family history of asthma or atopy (e.g. eczema, allergic rhinitis). The following symptoms may be triggered by pollens, dust, pets, exercise, infection, and allergens in the working environment:

- Wheeze
- Shortness of breath
- Chest tightness
- Cough

Nocturnal symptoms with sleep disturbance indicate severe asthma. Variability in airflow obstruction suggests the diagnosis of asthma such as:

- The peak flow rate shows a 20 per cent diurnal variation.
- The FEV1 will increase by > 15 per cent (and 200 ml) after a short acting β-agonist such as salbutamol.
- The FEV1 will increase by > 15 per cent (and 200 ml) after 14 days of prednisolone 30 mg od.
- The FEV1 will decrease by ≥ 15 per cent after six minutes of exercise.

Summary of Stepwise Management of Adult Asthma
(British Thoracic Society treatment guidelines 2004)

• Step 1	: Occasional use of short acting β_2-agonist. Go to step 2 if short acting β_2-agonist is used more than once a day.
• Step 2	: Add inhaled steroids: BDP 400 mcg /day.
• Step 3	: Add inhaled long-acting β-agonist (LABA). And increase inhaled steroids to BDP 800 mcg/day. If no response, stop LABA, add leukotriene RA *or* SR theophylline.
• Step 4	: Increased inhaled steroids to BDP 2000 mcg/day. Add leukotriene, *or* SR theophylline, *or* oral β_2-agonist.
• Step 5	: Add oral prednisolone and refer to specialist.

BDP = beclomethasone diproprionate
BDP or equivalent
Leukotriene RA = leukotriene receptor antagonist

REFERENCE

1. British guideline on the management of asthma: a national clinical guideline. British Thoracic Society and Scottish Intercollegiate Guidelines Network. Revised edition April 2004 (www.sign.ac.uk).

LINKS TO BOOK ONE

1. Case 39, page 121. Bronchial asthma.
2. Case 40, page 123. Obstructive lung disease.

Case 106

Cryptogenic Fibrosing Alveolitis

A 46-year-old farmer was referred to the respiratory clinic for investigation of breathlessness and a dry cough for the past three years. He was smoking 20 cigarettes a day. His General practitioner had been treating him for COPD. On examination, he was breathless at rest with an oxygen saturation of 88 per cent on room air. There was finger clubbing and crackles at the lower zone of both lungs. He was taking salbutamol 200 μg qds and becotide 200 μg puffs bd.

Hb	15.1 g/dl
WBC	$7.2 \times 10^9/l$
Platelets	$145 \times 10^9/l$
Na	134 mmol/l
K	5.2 mmol/l
Urea	7.2 mmol/ l
Creatinine	112 μmol/l
Glucose	5.2 mmol/l
PEFR	250 l/min
LFT	Normal
ANA	Negative
Rheumatoid factor	Negative
CXR	Irregular reticular shadowing in the lower zones

High-resolution CT chest showed a ground glass appearance and reticular shadowing in both lower zones.

The medical registrar arranged serology for microspora faeni and thermophilic actinomycetes and these were negative. PFT's were organised.

What is the likely diagnosis?

A. Extrinsic allergic alveolitis
B. Cryptogenic fibrosing alveolitis
C. COPD and chest infection
D. Interstitial fibrosis due to sarcoidosis
E. Bronchopulmonary aspergillosis

Answer (B)

DISCUSSION

Cryptogenic Fibrosing Alveolitis

Cryptogenic fibrosing alveolitis (CFA), or idiopathic pulmonary fibrosis, is a chronic progressive disease of the interstitial tissues of the lung with an unknown aetiology. The prevalence is 6 cases per 100,000 people. Each year the number of death from CFA in the UK is estimated to be more than 1,400. The male to female ratio is 2:1 and the mean age is 67 years. Inflammatory cells accumulate in the alveoli at an early stage, which gives rise to a ground glass appearance on the high resolution CT chest scan. Inflammation gives way to progressive fibrosis of the alveolar walls, distortion of the lung architecture and honeycombing.

Symptoms

- Shortness of breath is insidious and progressive.
- Dry cough
- Joint pains, weight loss, malaise.

Signs

- Finger clubbing is seen in 50 per cent of patients.
- Velcro like crackles at the end of inspiration is heard in the lower chest.
- Signs of right heart failure and pulmonary hypertension.

Investigations

- Exclude other causes of interstitial shadowing: asbestosis, drug induced pulmonary fibrosis, extrinsic allergic alveolitis (e.g. farmer's lung due to microspora faeni and thermophilic actinomycetes, or bird fancier's lung due to avian antigens),

sarcoidosis, infection (e.g. pneumocystis), cardiogenic pulmonary oedema, pulmonary eosinophilia, histiocytosis X, lymphomatoid granulomatosis and pulmonary alveolar proteinosis.
- Chest X-ray shows a diffuse reticular or reticulonodular infiltrate.
- High resolution CT chest: a ground glass appearance on CT suggests an active inflammatory response, which may respond to corticosteroids. End stage fibrotic change is untreatable.
- Arterial blood gases show hypoxia, but the $PaCO_2$ is normal until late stage.
- Lung function tests: spirometry shows a restrictive defect, small lung volumes and impaired diffusion capacity.
- Transbronchial lung biopsy or open lung biopsy.

Treatment

- Corticosteroids are more effective in those with a ground glass appearance on HR-chest CT and increased lymphocyte count in the bronchoalveolar lavage. A good response to prednisolone is seen in only 20 to 30 per cent of patients, but this is often short lived. In a typical regime, prednisolone in a dose of 0.5 mg/kg/day is given for 4 to 8 weeks and then tapered down over the next 3 months to 20 mg alternate days. The response to prednisolone is monitored by measuring the gas transfer coefficient (KCO) and TLC: generally a 15 per cent increase in these values is thought to be significant.
- Cytotoxics: azathioprine and cyclofosfamide have an anti-inflammatory action and steroid sparing effect.
- Antifibrotic agents: colchicine, D-penicillamine, pirfenidone and cyclosporin: the anti-fibrotic effect of these drugs has been disappointing.
- Gamma interferon inhibits inflammatory cytokine release and fibroblastic proliferation: only preliminary results are published.
- Domiciliary oxygen for hypoxic respiratory failure.
- Lung transplantation in selected patients (usually those who are under the age of 60 years where maximal medical therapy has failed). Single lung transplant has a 2-year survival rate of 60 to 80 per cent.

Prognosis

- The median survival is 3 to 5 years from onset of symptoms.
- Life expectancy is not altered by any of the currently available treatments.

LINKS TO BOOK ONE

1. Case 33, page 103. Wegener's granulomatosis.
2. Case 41, page 127. Restrictive lung disease.
3. Case 50, page 151. Amiodarone induced pulmonary disease.

Case 107

Pulmonary Embolism

A 40-year-old woman presented with sudden breathlessness. She was a life long non-smoker. There was no previous cardio-respiratory illness. She remained hypoxic despite 40 per cent oxygen therapy. The chest X- ray was normal. Her ventilation-perfusion lung scan is shown.

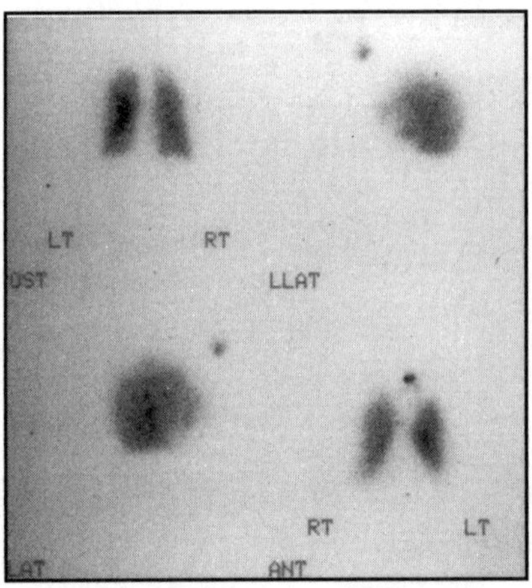

Ventilation scan

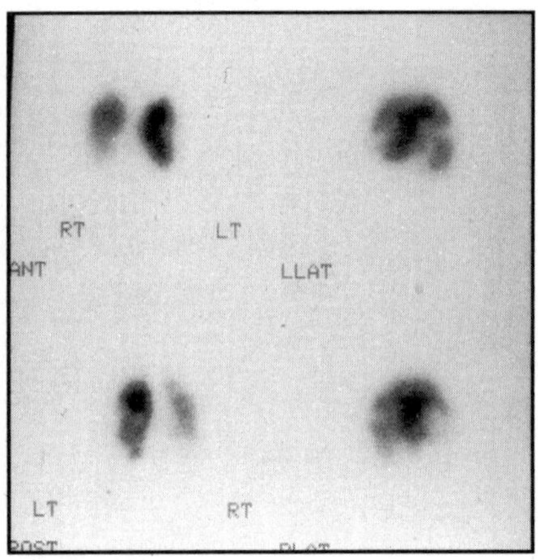

Perfusion scan

What other therapeutic measure is needed?

A. Aspirin
B. Warfarin
C. Low molecular weight heparin and oral warfarin
D. Intravenous antibiotic
E. Surgical embolectomy

Answer (C)

DISCUSSION

The perfusion scans show areas of non-perfusion with normal ventilation, consistent with pulmonary embolism (PE).

Pulmonary Embolism

The annual incidence of PE is 60 to 70 cases per 100,000 members of the UK population. Approximately 10 per cent of all hospital deaths are due to pulmonary embolism.

Clinical Probability Score for PE

Various clinical scoring systems have been used to assess the probability of PE, which can be combined with D-dimer test results for reducing the unnecessary demands on diagnostic imaging. The British Thoracic Society's guidelines for the management of suspected acute pulmonary embolism (2003) recommend all patients with possible PE should have clinical probability assessed and documented. The following clinical assessment scoring system is based on this report:

1. Is there breathlessness and/or tachypnoeic > 20/min?
   In the absence of these, pleuritic pain or haemoptysis is usually due to another cause.
2. Assess the clinical probability of PE by asking:
   a. Is another diagnosis *unlikely*?
   Review chest radiograph and ECG.

   b. Is there a major risk factor (e.g. recent immobility, major surgery, lower limb trauma or surgery, pregnancy or post partum, major medical illness, previous proven VTE)?
   High probability score = *both* (a) and (b)
   Intermediate probability score = (a) *or* (b)
   Low probability score = *neither* (a) or (b)

D-dimer assay

- Fibrinogen is cleaved by thrombin to produce fibrin monomers.
- Fibrin monomer strands are cross-linked by factor VIII.
- Plasmin lysis of these cross-linked fibrin strands generate D-dimer and other fragments (Figure 107.1).

- D-dimers can be measured using ELISA (e.g. Vidas), latex agglutination (e.g. MDA), and SimpliRED methods. SimpliRED uses a bispecific antibody with two different binding sites: one for red blood cells and the other for the D-dimer molecule. Agglutination of the patient's red blood cells occurs in the presence of elevated D-dimer levels.
- D-dimer assays have high sensitivity (> 90%), but poor specificity (45-68%), i.e. there are a substantial number of false positives, because elevated D-dimers are found in many other conditions including DIC, atrial fibrillation, intracardiac thrombi and left ventricular aneurysm. In practice only a *negative* D-dimer result is useful (see algorithm).
- A negative D-dimer test reliably excludes PE in-patients with low (SimpliRED, Vidas and MDA methods) or intermediate (Vidas, MDA) clinical probability; such patients do not require imaging for VTE (see BTS 2003 guidelines).
- The D-dimer test should not be performed in those with high clinical probability of PE (see BTS 2003 guidelines).

Diagnostic Imaging

PE can be confirmed using the following investigations:

- Ventilation-perfusion isotope lung scan. This method is not useful in people with underlying cardiopulmonary disease. Ventilation is measured using radiolabelled xenon. Perfusion is assessed by human albumin that has been radiolabelled with ^{99m}Technetium. In PE the isotope scan shows areas of non-perfusion that are not matched by defects in ventilation. Previous PE will also produce similar appearances. Indeterminate isotope lung scan results are common and require further diagnostic evaluation. A normal isotope scan reliably excludes PE. This method is not generally available outside normal working hours.
- Pulmonary angiography is the gold standard method, but seldom available.
- Spiral CT (i.e. computed tomographic pulmonary angiography, CTPA) is readily available, even outside normal working hours, and is the preferred initial investigation in non-massive PE. Clots in the main pulmonary trunk are easily documented, but subsegmental clots are less likely to be seen.

- The CTPA can show wedge shaped pulmonary infarcts and alternative causes for symptoms. CTPA is not affected by co-existing cardiorespiratory disease and can show acute changes in the right heart in massive PE such as dilatation of the right ventricle and interventricular septal displacement.
- Doppler leg ultrasound. In a patient with deep venous thrombosis (DVT) co-existing with possible PE, leg ultrasound can be the initial investigation. Evidence for a DVT may help in the decision to anticoagulate in someone with an equivocal isotope lung scan result. A single negative leg ultrasound does not reliably exclude proximal DVT.

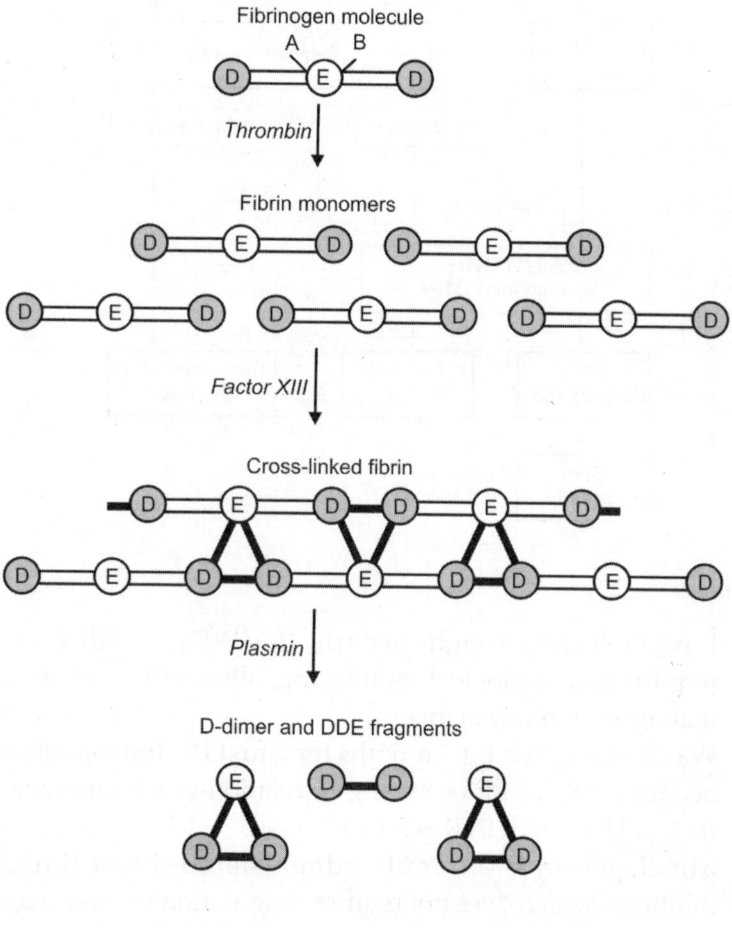

Figure 107.1: Formation of fibrin and its lysis to D-dimers and other fragments

Table 107.1: Algorithm for suspected non-massive pulmonary embolism

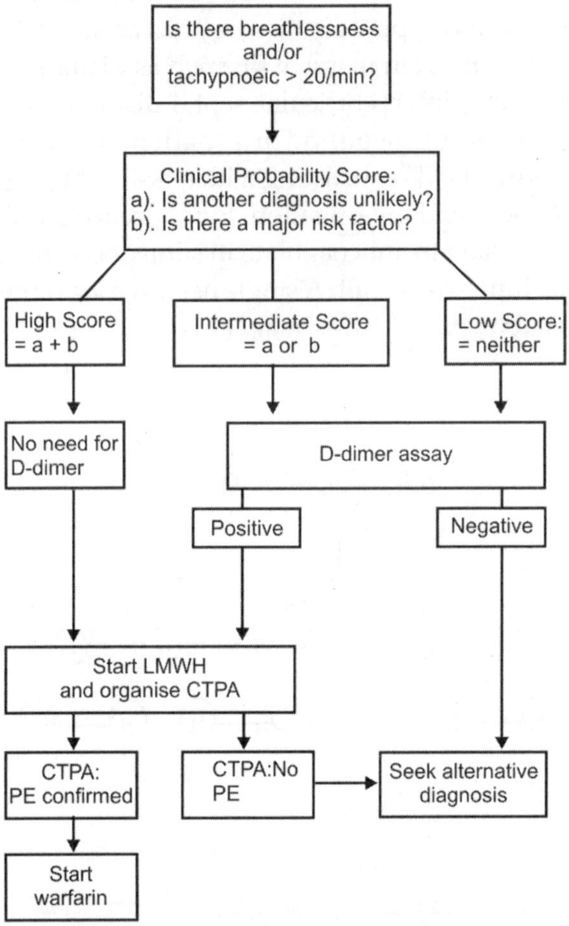

Treatment

- Low molecular weight heparin (LMWH), which does not require haematological monitoring, allows PE patients to be managed as out-patients.
- Warfarin is given for 3 months for a first PE, but 6 weeks may be sufficient for PE occurring in relation to a temporary risk factor. The target INR is 2 to 3
- Ximelagatran is an orally administered direct thrombin inhibitor, which does not require coagulation monitoring, and looks promising in the future treatment of PE or DVT.
- Thrombolysis is the first line treatment for massive PE (= associated with circulatory collapse): alteplase is better than

streptokinase as it does not exacerbate hypotension. If cardiac arrest is imminent 50 mg IV bolus of alteplase can be given. Fragmentation of the thrombus using a right heart catheter and IVC filter are only available in a few centres.

REFERENCES

1. British Thoracic Society guidelines for the management of suspected acute pulmonary embolism. Thorax 2003; 58: 470-484 (www.brit-thoracic.org.uk)
2. Lip GYH and Lowe GDO. Fibrin D-dimer: a useful clinical marker of thrombogenesis. Clinical Science 1995;89:205-14.
3. British Thoracic Society. Optimum duration of anticoagulation for deep vein thrombosis and pulmonary embolism. Lancet 1992;340:873-6.
4. Frances CW et al. Comparison of ximelagatan with warfarin for the prevention of venous thromboembolism after total knee replacement. NEJM 2003;349:1703-12.

LINKS TO BOOK ONE

1. Case 26, page 75. Heparin induced thrombocytopenia.
2. Case 28, page 85. Thrombophilia.
3. Case 99, page 341. Pulmonary embolism.

Case 108

Arterial Blood Gases (Metabolic Alkalosis)

A 64-year-old man with vomiting has the following arterial blood gas results taken on room air.

pH	7.51
PaO_2	8.68 kPa
$PaCO_2$	6.57 kPa
HCO_3	38.9 mmol/l

What is the most likely diagnosis?

A. Metabolic alkalosis
B. Respiratory acidosis
C. Combined metabolic and respiratory acidosis
D. Uncompensated respiratory acidosis
E. Metabolic acidosis

Answer (A)

DISCUSSION

There is an alkalotic pH (= 7.51) and raised serum bicarbonate (HCO_3 = 38.9 mmol/l). The high $PaCO_2$ is compensatory.

Tips in Arterial Blood Gas Interpretation

1. Look at the pH: decide whether it is an:
   acidosis (pH < 7.35)
   or
   alkalosis (pH > 7.45)
2. Look at the $PaCO_2$ and HCO_3:
   - acidotic pH + High $PaCO_2$ = respiratory acidosis
   - alkalotic pH + High $PaCO_2$ = the high CO_2 is compensatory
   - alkalotic pH + High HCO_3 = metabolic alkalosis
   - acidotic pH + High HCO_3 = the high HCO_3 is compensatory

Causes of Metabolic Alkalosis

- Vomiting or nasogastric suction.
- Diarrhoea
- Diuretic therapy
- Potassium depletion (e.g. excess mineralocorticoids: Conn's syndrome, liquorice intake, Cushing's syndrome).
- Antacids (Milk-alkali syndrome: hypercalcaemia from milk with excess antacid).
- Excess IV sodium bicarbonate, sodium lactate, sodium citrate and sodium gluconate.
- Post-hypercapnia alkalosis (due to too rapid correction of elevated $PaCO_2$ with mechanical ventilation i.e. before renal bicarbonaturia can remove the excess HCO_3)

LINKS TO BOOK ONE

1. Case 47, page 144. Chronic compensated respiratory acidosis.
2. Case 53, page 165. Metabolic alkalosis.
3. Case 54, page 167. Acute respiratory alkalosis.
4. Case 90, page 307. Type 1 respiratory failure.
5. Case 93, page 319. Type 2 respiratory failure.

Case 109

Unilateral Hyperlucency

What is the abnormality on this chest X-ray?

A. Left mastectomy
B. Emphysema
C. MacLeods's syndrome
D. Left pneumonectomy
E. Collapse of the left lung

Answer (A)

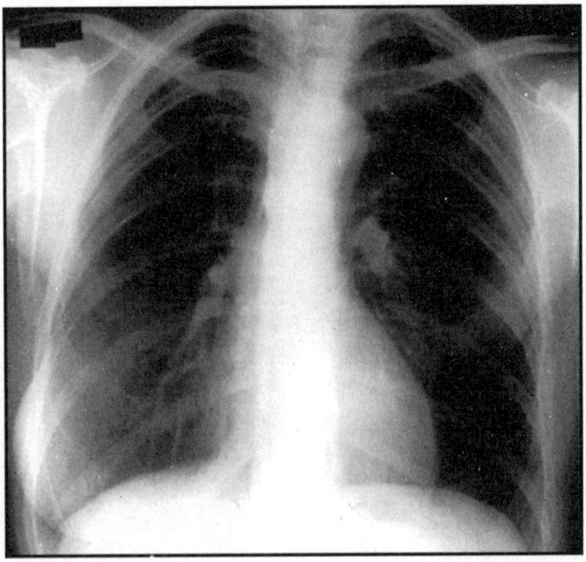

DISCUSSION

Differential Diagnosis of Unilateral Hyperlucency

The possible causes of increased lucency of one lung are:

Pathology outside the thorax

- Absent breast (including mastectomy).
- Absent chest wall muscle (including Poland's syndrome: absent pectoralis major, hypoplastic arm and syndactyly).

Lung disease

- Pneumothorax
- Emphysema
- Bullous lung disease
- Obstructive emphysema (large lungs): due to bronchial obstruction (including tumour, foreign body, mucous plugging in asthma, hilar lymph nodes, enlarged left atrium in mitral stenosis).
- Compensatory expansion (e.g. following collapse of the left lower lobe)
- Pulmonary embolism (asymmetrical oligaemia).
- Macleod's syndrome: viral infection in early life leading to failure of normal lung size development (see below).
- Congenital: congenitally absent or hypoplastic pulmonary artery.

Technical problems

- Over penetration (usually causes bilateral hyperlucency).
- Rotation

Apparent hyperlucency

- The other lung is diseased and more densely opacified (e.g. due to supine pleural effusion). In this situation the normal lung will appear comparatively hyperlucent.

Swyer-James-MacCleod's Syndrome

Sometimes simply referred to as MacCleod's syndrome. Viral bronchiolitis in childhood leads to failure of the lung to develop normally. A whole lung or just one lobe may be affected. Alveoli numbers never reach the adult number. The pulmonary arterial supply is also diminished. Later in adult life, the affected lung may develop panacinar emphysema, recurrent infections and bronchiectasis. Most cases are asymptomatic and the abnormality is picked up as a result of a routine chest X-ray. Radiologically, the abnormally hyperlucent lung may be normal in size (or smaller with deviation of the mediastinum towards it) and contain fewer pulmonary vessels markings. During expiration, air trapping in the abnormal lung may occur and cause the mediastinum to move across to the opposite side.

Case 110

Mycoplasma Pneumoniae

A 32-year-old teacher developed a low-grade fever, sore throat, and dry cough for three days. She attended the A and E department on New Years Eve. One week ago, her General Practitioner started her on amoxicillin 500 mg tds. Two days later she became more unwell with left sided pleuritic pain and presented to the local A and E. She was pyrexial (39.2° Celsius) and tachypnoeic with a respiratory rate 30/minute. The SaO_2 was 92 per cent on room air. Her chest-ray showed patchy consolidation in the left lower zone. The registrar noticed the patient had very cold and blue hands. Cold agglutinins were markedly positive.

What is the most likely organism of her chest infection?

A. *Streptococcus pneumoniae*
B. *Haemophilus influenzae*
C. *Staphylococcus aureus*
D. *Influenza pneumonia*
E. *Mycoplasma pneumoniae*

Answer (E)

DISCUSSION

***Mycoplasma pneumoniae* is suggested by:**

- Slow onset
- Upper respiratory tract symptoms, such as sore throat, earache
- Young age
- Cold agglutinins: haemolytic anaemia, Raynaud's phenomena or acrocyanosis

Community Acquired Pneumonia

The incidence of community-acquired pneumonia (CAP) is 6 per 1,000 people in the age group 16-59 and 34 per 1,000 in those aged 75 years or more. About one third of patients will need to be admitted to hospital and one in ten will require admission to an intensive care unit. The overall mortality from pneumonia is 5 to 10 per cent for hospital in-patients. The severity of pneumonia is given by the CURB-65 score:

- C = Confusion
- U = Urea > 7 mmol/l
- R = Respiratory rate ≥ 30/minute
- B = Blood pressure (systolic BP < 90 mmHg or diastolic BP < 60 mmHg)
- Age ≥ 65 years

Note: Each of the above items has a score of 1.

*CURB-65 score**	*Mortality*	*Treatment Option*
0 to 1	Low (1.5%)	Probably suitable for home treatment #
2	Intermediate (9.2%)	Hospital in-patient treatment *Or* Hospital out-patient supervised treatment
3 or more	High (22%)	Manage in hospital as severe pneumonia. Assess for ITU if CURB = 4 or 5

Notes:

* Lim WS et al 2003

The decision to admit or treat at home will also depend on social factors – hospital admission may be needed for frail, isolated elderly patients with co-morbidity – or where compliance is unpredictable.

Mycoplasma Pneumoniae

Mycoplasma pneumoniae is the causative organism in 10-20 per cent cases of community-acquired pneumonia. (Note: *Streptococcus pneumoniae* is the most common pathogen and accounts for 50% of cases). *Mycoplasma* infection tends to affect the young, with outbreaks occurring very 4 to 8 years in schools and colleges. It is spread by inhalation of infected secretions. Some infected individuals are asymptomatic. The incubation period is about three weeks. The onset is gradual with a dry cough, which can persist for several weeks, fever, sore throat, earache, headache, and malaise. The chest X-ray findings are non-specific, such as patchy consolidation, linear atelectasis, and pleural effusion. Cold agglutinins may occur in

50 to 75 per cent of patients, but haemolytic anaemia is uncommon. Other systemic complications may also have an immunological basis and include myopericarditis, hepatitis, thrombocytopenia, Guillain-Barré syndrome, lymphocytic meningitis and erythema multiforme. The diagnosis is made serologically or by detection of *Mycoplasma* RNA using the polymerise chain reaction method. There is usually a complete recovery following treatment with a macrolide antibiotic (erythromycin or clarithromycin).

Community Acquired Pneumonia

The microorganisms are usually one of the following:

- *Streptococcus pneumoniae*
- *Mycoplasma pneumoniae*
- *Chlamydia pneumoniae*
- Viral (e.g. influenza)
- *Haemophilus influenzae*
- *Staphylococcus aureus* (especially after influenza)
- *Legionella pneumophila*

The appropriate antibiotic regimes are:

- Amoxicillin 500 mg – 1g tds, or Clarithromycin if allergic to penicillin
- Add Clarithromycin 500 mg bd if atypical organisms suspected (Atypical organisms include *Mycoplasma, Chlamydia, Legionella*)
- Severely ill patients: Cefuroxime 1.5 g tds, or Cefotaxime + Clarithromycin 500 mg bd
- IV ciprofloxacin 500 mg bd + benzylpenicillin 1.2g qds is an alternative regime in severe pneumonia

REFERENCE

1. Lim WS et al. Defining community acquired pneumonia severity on presentation to hospital: an international derivation and validation study. Thorax 2003;58;377-82.
2. BTS Guidelines for the management of community acquired pneumonia in adults. Thorax 2001;56(Suppl. 4):iv 1-64.

LINKS TO BOOK ONE

1. Case 63, page 199. Hypogammaglobulinaemia.

Case 111

Abnormal Chest X-ray (Calcified Thyroid Nodule/cyst)

This patient has atrial fibrillation and weight loss. She was short of breath at rest. There were no symptoms of cough, chest pain, and haemoptysis. She was a non-smoker. The chest X-ray was obtained (see below). Bronchoscopy and cytology were negative.

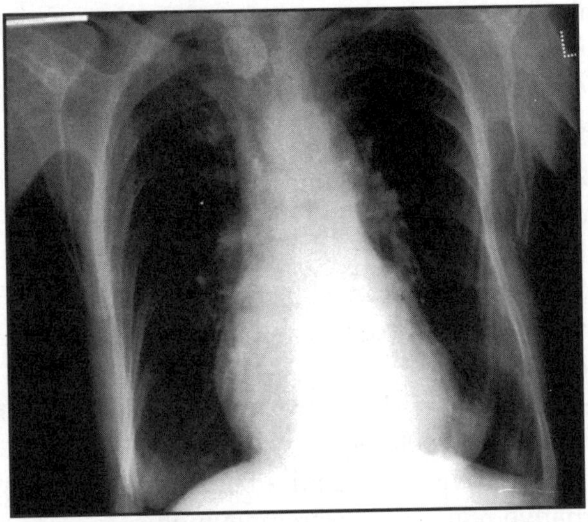

What are the next most important two diagnostic measures?

A. Thyroid isotope scan
B. Thyroid function tests
C. Thyroid auto-antibodies
D. Mediastinoscopy
E. Surgical exploration of the mediastinum
F. Ambulatory ECG monitoring
G. Echocardiography
H. Gastroscopy

Answers (A, B)

DISCUSSION

This patient has a calcified lesion in the lower neck and upper mediastinum. The most likely diagnosis is a calcified thyroid nodule or cyst. An ultrasound will distinguish between solid and cystic lesions. Larger lesions with tracheal compression, including those with a significant retrosternal component, are best evaluated using CT or MRI scans. Cystic thyroid lesions are usually benign, but there are exceptions (see below). The question of malignancy in a thyroid nodule or cyst cannot be reliably settled without diagnostic aspiration. Atrial fibrillation and weight loss in this patient suggest hyperthyroidism, which can be confirmed by thyroid function tests and the radioisotope scan may show a hyperfunctioning "hot" nodule. Thyroid auto-antibodies (such as thyroid peroxidase, TPO) provide no useful indication as to whether a thyroid nodule is benign or malignant.

Thyroid nodules

- Thyroid nodules, which may be single or multiple, can be demonstrated in 50 per cent of the population using high resolution ultrasound.
- Only five per cent of thyroid nodules detected by ultrasound are clinically palpable.
- At postmortem 50 per cent of patients who have clinically normal thyroid glands are found to have thyroid nodules and five per cent harbour thyroid malignancy.
- Thyroid cancer is rare and accounts for only one per cent of all malignancies. In the UK there are 1,100 new cases of thyroid cancer each year.
- The challenge is to identify the small number of thyroid cancers among the many who present with benign thyroid nodules.

Radiographs

Plain X-rays may show the following signs:

- A rim of egg shell calcification suggests a benign nodule.
- Stippled calcification suggests carcinoma.
- Calcified metastastic deposits occur in medullary thyroid carcinoma.
- Pulmonary and bony metastases from thyroid carcinoma.
- Displacement of the trachea or tracheal stenosis can occur in both benign and malignant goitre.

Radioisotope imaging of the thyroid

This can be performed with either ^{123}Iodine or ^{99m}Technetium (see Table 111.1 for differences in methodology).

- Radioisotope scintigraphic scans may reveal multiple nodules, retrosternal goitre, ectopic functioning thyroid tissue, and functioning metastases from thyroid carcinoma.
- Thyroidal uptake of a radioactive tracer such ^{123}Iodine or ^{99m}Technetium at a standard time after administration provides an indication of thyroid function. Thyrotoxicosis can be subdivided into high uptake and low uptake (see Table 111.2).
- Radioisotope studies cannot reliably distinguish between malignant nodules (which are generally non-functioning and do not take up radioisotope) from benign nodules (which are generally "hot" due to increased uptake).
- In one series malignancy was found in four per cent of hot nodules and 16 per cent of cold nodules.

Thyroid ultrasound

Ultrasound can detect cystic lesions > 2mm and solid nodules > 3mm.

- Ultrasound show thyroid nodules are very common and occur in 50 per cent of the population.
- Thyroid cysts are produced by degeneration of an existing

Table 111.1: Comparison of ^{123}Iodine radioiodine and ^{99m}Technetium thyroid scans

	^{123}Iodine	*^{99m}Technetium*
Half life	13 hours	6 hours
Dose	100-200 μCi (3.7-7.4 MBq*)	1-10 μCi (37-370 MBq)
Main indications	For scintigraphy (i.e. the visualization of thyroid anatomy, recording of functioning ('hot') and non-functioning ('cold') nodules.	For rapid measurement of thyroid uptake at 30 min (i.e. the trapping of 99m-Tc radioisotope) and evaluation of thyroid function. Technetium is not organified and rapidly leaks out of the thyroid gland.
Main advantages and disadvantages	* Relatively expensive * Generated by cyclotron and less readily available	* Cheap * Readily available * Not sensitive for nodules < 5 mm
	*MBq = Mega Bequerel	

Table 111.2: Hyperthyroidism according to differences in thyroid radioisotope uptake

Hyperthyroidism with high uptake	*Hyperthyroidism with low uptake*
Graves' disease	Thyroiditis e.g. subacute thyroiditis, postpartum thyroiditis.
Toxic single adenoma (Plummer's disease)	Iodine excess (i.e. Jod Basedow phenomenon) e.g. amiodarone.
Toxic multinodular goitre	Factitious thyrotoxicosis due to the surreptitious intake of thyroxine (thyroglobulin is characteristically undetectable in these patients).
Hydatidiform mole (produces HCG which has TSH like properties)	Hamburger thyrotoxicosis (due to beef thyroid tissue ingestion)
Pituitary TSH producing adenoma and inappropriate TSH secretion	
Metastatic thyroid cancer (multiple skeletal foci of increased uptake)	
Struma ovarii (ovarian teratoma containing hyperactive thyroid tissue with increased uptake in the pelvis)	

thyroid nodule.

- Solid or mixed solid-cystic lesions are more likely to be malignant, but not all cystic lesions are harmless. In one series 6 per cent of cystic lesions were malignant and 94 per cent were benign.

Diagnostic fine needle aspiration

Needle aspiration of thyroid nodules and cysts is recommended to rule out malignancy. Ultrasound guided aspiration is used for non-palpable nodules and for alcohol ablation of autonomous hyper-functioning nodules. Aspiration is also a curative procedure for benign cysts. Recurrent thyroid cysts can be treated with ultrasound guided injection of alcohol or tetracycline.

LINKS TO BOOK ONE

1. Case 8, page 22. Thyroid autoantibodies.
2. Case 30, page 93. Sick euthyroid syndrome.
3. Case 36, page 111. Amiodarone induced thyroid disease.

Case 112

Abnormal Chest X-ray (Chickenpox Pneumonia)

This chest X-ray is taken for an insurance medical examination and belongs to an asymptomatic young woman. It shows multiple bilateral small calcified nodules.

What is the diagnosis?

A. Chickenpox pneumonia
B. Miliary tuberculosis
C. Previous influenza infection
D. Idiopathic haemosiderosis
E. Bronchiectasis

Answer (A)

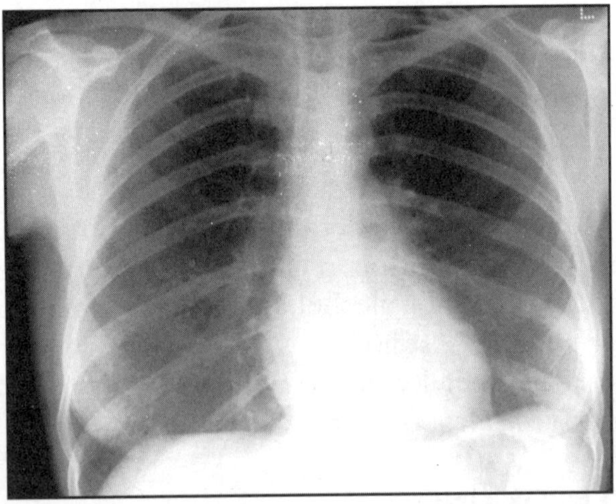

DISCUSSION

This chest X-ray shows diffuse tiny calcifications in the lung fields in an otherwise healthy individual, which is compatible with the diagnosis of previous chickenpox pneumonia.

Complications of Chickenpox (Varicella-Zoster Virus)

- Varicella pneumonia. This is more common in teenagers, adults, smokers, those with underlying lung disease, and the last trimester of pregnancy. It can be complicated by ARDS. The treatment is IV aciclovir and supportive measures. Healing of the lung occurs with fine nodular calcification.
- Herpes zoster (shingles). After an attack of chickenpox in the childhood, the varicella-zoster virus can remain dormant in the dorsal root ganglion. Reactivation of the virus later on in life produces the painfully blistering rash of herpes zoster, particularly if there is impaired immunity (e.g. malignancy, HIV, cytotoxic therapy, and corticosteroid medication). About one in five immunocompetent people at some time in their life will develop shingles. Involvement of the V cranial nerve produces ophthalmic herpes, which can lead to corneal scarring. Geniculate herpes is involvement of the VII nerve in the middle ear and produces the Ramsey Hunt syndrome, which presents as facial palsy with a vesicular rash on the pinna.
- Individuals who are not already immune can catch chickenpox from patients with shingles. Shingles is infectious from the *onset of the rash until all the scabs have crusted.* The period of infectivity in chickenpox is *4 days before and 5 days after the rash starts.*
- Post herpetic neuralgia (PHN) is the pain that sometimes follows the resolution and healing of the acute herpes zoster rash. It is defined as pain that persists more than 6 weeks after the development of rash. The PHN is rare in people under the age of 50 years, but the risk increases with advancing age. The PHN can develop in 10 to 40 per cent of elderly people with shingles. Early antiviral therapies given within three days of onset may prevent PHN (e.g. valaciclovir) or reduce its duration and severity (e.g. aciclovir). The pain of PHN can be severely distressing, but will gradually subside, although 30 per cent are still symptomatic after one year. Tricyclic antidepressants (e.g. amitriptyline), anticonvulsants (e.g. gabapentin) and nerve blocks may help.
- Contralateral ischaemic stroke in young adults due to cerebral vasculitis has been described after an attack of ophthalmic herpes zoster.

- Acute cerebellar ataxia
- Encephalitis
- Guillain-Barré syndrome
- Reye's syndrome (encephalopathy and fatty liver) can occur when aspirin is given to children with chickenpox.
- Thrombocytopenia
- Myocarditis

Congenital Varicella Syndrome

- As chickenpox is rare in adults, its occurrence in pregnancy is unusual.
- In the UK 17 out of 20 pregnant women have already had chickenpox as a child and are immune. The remaining three out of 20 pregnant women have not previously had chickenpox.
- The lack of immunity can be confirmed by the absence of antibodies to the varicella-zoster virus. These women can be given varicella-zoster immunoglobulin within 10 days of exposure.
- Varicella infection during the fist trimester of pregnancy can lead to stillbirth or the child may be born with the following congenital defects: cicatrical skin lesions, hypoplasia of limbs and digits, mental retardation, seizures, deafness, blindness (due to chorioretinitis, cataracts, and other ocular lesions).

REFERENCE

1. Gilden DH, et al. Neurologic complications of the reactivation of varicella-zoster virus. NEJM 2000;342:635-45.
2. PILS leaflets: L269 chickenpox in adults and L270 chickenpox, shingles and pregnancy (www.prodigy.nhs.uk/ClinicalGuidance).

Index

A

B

C

G

H

I

J

K

L

M